Silence

To Mum and Dad,
gone, but always in my heart

An Hachette UK Company
www.hachette.co.uk

First published in Great Britain
in 2020 by Gaia, an imprint of
Octopus Publishing Group Ltd
Carmelite House
50 Victoria Embankment
London EC4Y 0DZ
www.octopusbooks.co.uk

Distributed in the US by
Hachette Book Group
1290 Avenue of the Americas
4th and 5th Floors
New York, NY 10104

Distributed in Canada by
Canadian Manda Group
664 Annette St.
Toronto, Ontario, Canada M6S 2C8

ISBN 978-1-85675-420-0

A CIP catalogue record for this book is available
from the British Library.

Printed and bound in China.

10 9 8 7 6 5 4 3 2 1

Publishing Director: Stephanie Jackson
Senior Editor: Pollyanna Poulter
Art Director: Yasia Williams
Senior Production Controller:
   Allison Gonsalves
Copy Editor: Caroline Taggart
Proofreader: Alison Wormleighton
Indexer: MFE Editorial
Designer: Leonardo Collina

Silence

Harnessing the restorative
power of silence in
a noisy world

Joanna Nylund

CONTENTS

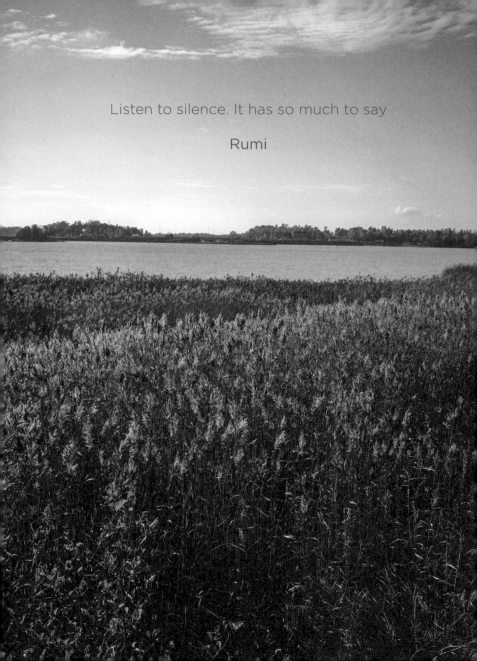

Listen to silence. It has so much to say

Rumi

FOREWORD

For some years now, I have seen my capacity to concentrate dwindle with every hour spent mindlessly scrolling social media feeds. I have started, and quit, another job in an open-plan office after just not being able to take the noise anymore. I have felt my blood pressure and stress levels rise due to the sheer amount of input, auditory and visual, that I let myself get bombarded with every day. I feel mentally tired, overwhelmed and more than a little confused. Something has to give. But what? And more importantly – how?

The book you are holding in your hands is an attempt to answer those questions. It has been informed by a yearning to recapture a core of inner stillness that I remember from childhood. A desire to regain my ability to focus single-mindedly on something, not just for minutes but for hours on end. I would like to feel calm, collected and in charge of my time. These are some of the reasons why I've decided to go searching for something that, if not exactly lost, has fallen right to the bottom of my list of daily priorities: silence.

We are all well aware that there is a problem with the pace and intensity of modern life. There is a myriad of books and articles trying to help us cope. Is this another one? Perhaps. But silence is neither gimmicky nor new. It is a natural resource that has always been available to us to varying degrees, but it wouldn't be an exaggeration to claim it is now endangered in a way that it has never been before.

In its broadest sense, silence encompasses everything that makes things go quiet inside. A book about silence is necessarily also a book about its opposite number, noise. I will look at the kind of noise we see as well as the kind we hear. I will investigate the role silence has played in our cultural history, and talk to people with different experiences of silence to find out what they have discovered. I will also expose myself to different kinds of silence and try my best not to shy away from asking some hard questions about the way I lead my life.

Most importantly, perhaps, I will look high and low for ways of allowing all of us to increase the amount of silence in our lives – without moving to a hermit's cave.

So, *shh* – let's begin.

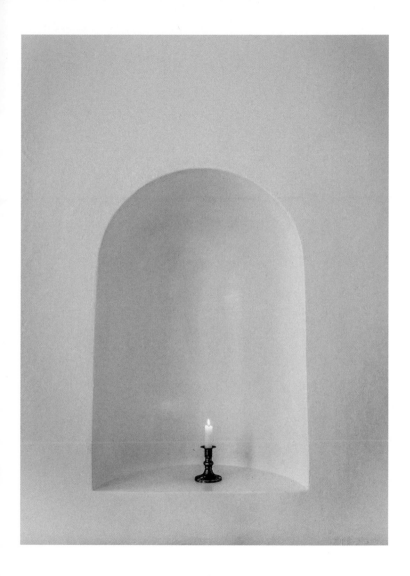

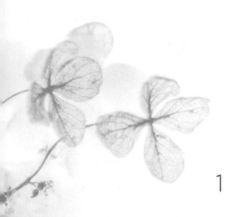

1

THE SOUND OF SILENCE

A fool is known by his speech,
a wise man by his silence

Pythagoras

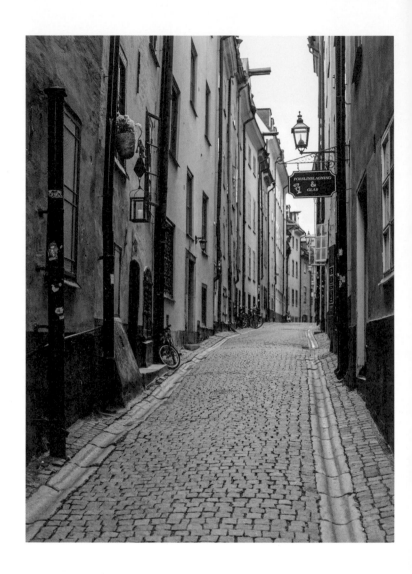

A SILENT ENIGMA
SEARCHING FOR A HIDDEN GEM

In a noisy world, silence is an increasingly depleted natural resource. But is silence more than just the absence of sound? And is there such a thing as absolute silence? Aside from external silence, we also need silence within us. What does that look like and how do we achieve it? And, despite the obvious connection between silence and solitude, can we experience silence without having to leave everything behind?

The first thing to be said about silence? That there really is no such thing.

As I write this in my study at home, I can hear the elevator running. The building next door is having its balconies replaced, and for weeks now the inescapable sound of a drill working its way through concrete has resonated through our otherwise reasonably quiet neighbourhood. In the distance I can hear the steady swishing of cars on the motorway: a wall of noise much like running water, but noise nevertheless. Even so, my home is a place I always describe as quiet, and by any urban standards it certainly is.

It was only a few years ago that I began reflecting on noise sensitivity. I'm one of those people who painstakingly go through the list of available ring tones in order to find the most discreet one, only to leave my phone on silent anyway.

I turn down the volume on the TV as soon as I turn it on. I love music, but detest having it on in the background for the purpose of creating an ambience; it makes me feel manipulated. With all this in mind I would describe myself as probably more sensitive to sound than most people – however, stopping short of requiring a soundproof bunker for my peace of mind.

One thing is clear, though: I've become more sensitive over the years. My siblings and I used to laugh at our mother when she would cover her ears while watching a thriller on TV, and now I do the same. It is always the sounds, not the images, that make me jump. Sometimes even the doorbell ringing causes my heartbeat to soar, and topping the list of unpleasant sensations is loud, unexpected noise.

This stands in sharp contrast to our downstairs neighbours, whose lives seem to be conducted with the volume turned up to the max. Normal everyday exchanges are shouted rather than spoken. Doors are slammed. They even *walk* loudly, heels thudding against the floor. Somehow it was no surprise that when they got a dog it would turn out to be a howler. In case all this makes me sound like that neighbour from hell who insists on finding fault with everything, let me quickly add that they remain unaware of my feelings regarding their, hmm, lifestyle. (I write about them instead.)

Nevertheless, my involuntary field studies lead me to believe that, in some families, quiet is an unknown phenomenon, and I dare say they are better equipped to deal with the modern world than I am.

A friend who is an entrepreneur is showing me around his company office. It is open-plan with large screens dominating the walls. He enthusiastically mentions that music is played throughout the day. *How absolutely horrible*, I think to myself. But I say nothing. Aside from not wanting to hurt his feelings, I feel a little embarrassed about my inability to tolerate noise. It makes me feel outdated. Surely we are supposed to go with the flow these days? Aren't we meant to be dynamic, multi-tasking beings in a constant, creative give-and-take?

It might work for my friend and a few other extremely social people, but for the rest of us the gap between ideal and painful reality is as big as ever. Studies now show that the sensory input and distractions that come from sharing office space actually tend to reduce efficiency and increase stress levels. In the name of that favourite corporate buzzword, *synergy* (read: saving money on space), we persist, however. But at what cost? Only time will tell.

DEAFENING SILENCE
IS QUIET REALLY ALL THAT PEACEFUL?

Space is reportedly silent. The planets make no noise as they revolve on their axis and around the Sun. But as soon as we enter space to hear this silence for ourselves, noise interferes: if not the creaking of our space suits and the crackle of radio communications, then ultimately the sound of our heartbeat and the rushing of blood in our veins.

Case in point: composer John Cage once visited an anechoic chamber, a soundproof room built to absorb all noise created within it, and was disappointed to hear two notes, one high and one low. Convinced that the chamber didn't work, he asked the technician what these sounds were. He was told that the high note was his nervous system in operation and the low note the sound of his blood circulation. This persuaded Cage that absolute silence does not exist and inspired his famous composition 4'33", often known as "four minutes of silence" but actually consisting of the noise the audience makes while the piece is "played": coughing, shuffling papers, moving about.

Most of us do not have access to an anechoic chamber, but may still have experienced the unnerving effect of near-absolute silence. Aside from possibly hearing bodily functions we never otherwise notice, there is evidence to suggest that, in extreme silence, our brains manufacture their own noise. Sometimes there is a ringing in the ears

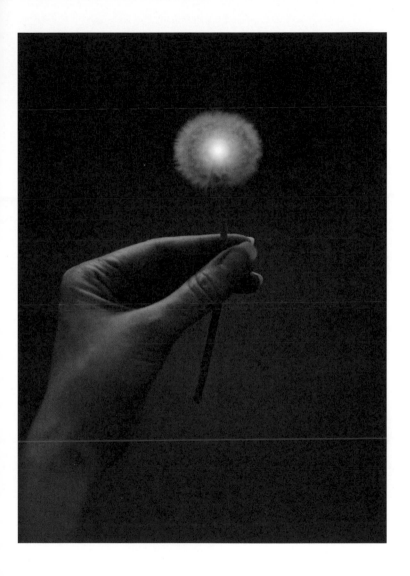

that resembles tinnitus. It is also possible to "hear" noise that isn't actually there, like a hallucination (just think how easy it is to "hear" music in your mind sometimes). What creates this effect is still uncertain, but scientists believe it is possible that our auditory memory plays recordings back to us, as it were, as a way of coping with the lack of sensory input that deep silence brings. A completely silent world seems to make our brains nervous.

Without floating off into space, it is still possible to test the effect of near-absolute silence. To help us we have two substances with built-in soundproofing: sand and snow.

"The strange thing about the desert," says my husband, who has been sleeping on its sand during a stay in Jordan, "is that although you are in this vast expanse, the feeling is almost of being indoors. The silence is so intense that it seemed I could hear it."

The highly insulating quality of sand effectively stops sound waves in their tracks. No wonder the desert has always acted like a magnet for people seeking an escape from the hubbub.

In my corner of the world – Finland – children build snow caves to play in and adults build snow hotels for tourists. Remembering the cosy but slightly odd feeling of sitting inside a snow cave as a child, I speak to a woman who has spent a night in a hotel made entirely from snow and ice (it melts and is rebuilt every year).

"We live in the countryside, so I'm used to nights being very silent," she says. "But this was different. Not only did the snow insulate us from any outside noise, we also happened to be the only guests staying at the hotel that night. When I lay down to sleep, the only noise I could hear was my own breathing. It sounded so loud."

She hastens to assure me the experience was strange but positive. My guess is that someone less used to silence could also find it eerie.

On the whole, complete silence is apparently not something we thrive in. Good to know, but our challenge is really something else: finding even five minutes of moderate silence in a day and thriving in them.

Silence is a true friend who never betrays

Confucius

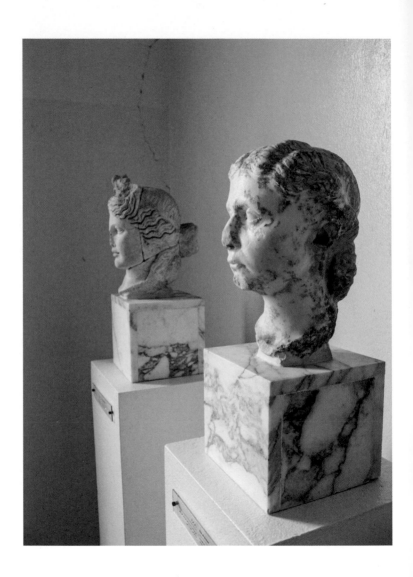

SILENCE FOR THE EYES
A PROBLEM BIGGER THAN NOISE

I've created a fairly silent working environment for myself, but the silence I lack the most is doubtless of another kind. Who doesn't know the feeling of turning off the lights at night in order to go to sleep, only to be inundated by a flood of images? Technically they are silent, but they still scramble our brains to the extent that they might as well be making noise. We want to *hear ourselves think*, we say, and what stops us these days is just as likely to be visual noise as the audible kind.

Considering the sheer amount of distractions available, silence is an increasingly unknown phenomenon to many people. We are stuck in a vicious circle: the less used to silence we become, the more we will fear it – and the harder it will be for us to face it. Could it be that we are now distracting ourselves to the point where quiet introspection is virtually non-existent?

It matters little that my surroundings are silent if my mind is loud. External silence is often necessary in order to create internal silence, but it can't do the job on its own. And, interestingly, when my mind is silent, my threshold for withstanding audible noise becomes a lot higher.

SILENCE VS SOLITUDE
IS IT NECESSARY TO WITHDRAW
FROM THE WORLD?

There are many great books about silence out there, with many wise thinkers down the ages ruminating on silence and the pursuit of it. With a few exceptions they have one thing in common: these seekers of quiet have literally gone to great lengths to find it. Leaving the world and its noises behind, they have ventured into deserts, scaled the highest peaks and sailed faraway seas. We can learn a lot from their experiences, but when it comes to finding silence for ourselves in the midst of our busy urban lives, these accounts do not offer much in the way of practical help.

Do silence and solitude always go together? It stands to reason that solitude is a great help, but I'm willing to wager the whole of this book on the belief that it can't be a prerequisite for silence. The majority of the world's population resides in cities. Most of us don't have the luxury of checking out of our daily lives. The real challenge, then, lies in finding pockets of silence *where we are*, to sustain us in the life that is ours. This is no easy task. But I believe it is necessary in order to harness the powerful impact that silence could have on us.

If, however, we were given the chance to have a one-off experience of silence in solitude, maybe it could prove a stepping stone to increased silence in our daily lives.

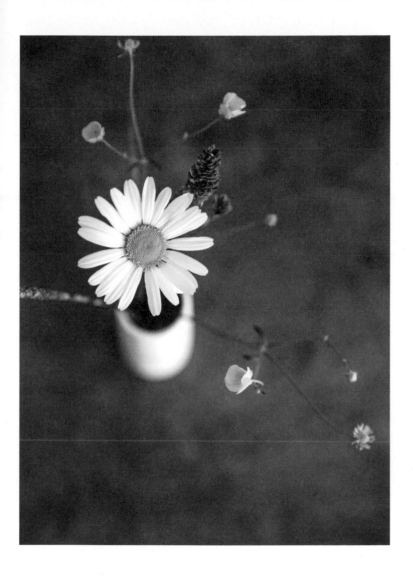

Around the World in Silence – Lessons from the Extreme

Author and mountaineer Geordie Stewart is someone who often chooses to expose himself to periods of silence and solitude. In 2011, aged 22, he became the youngest Briton ever to have scaled the Seven Summits – the highest mountain on each of the seven continents. More recently, he explored the world from a much lower vantage point: his bicycle saddle. I discussed with him his approach to silence and solitude, whether at home or away.

Geordie, you chose to cycle around the world by yourself, something that you knew would expose you to lengthy periods of solitude and silence. When you were setting out, how did you feel about that prospect?

I knew solitude would be an unavoidable reality when venturing alone on a bike across several continents. But I never felt fearful about the prospect, nor did I see it as an insurmountable obstacle. Instead, it was something I craved, was fascinated by and wanted to embrace.

Care to name a really memorable, positive experience of silence? How has silence challenged you?

In May 2010, I returned to the UK after my failed attempt to summit Everest having turned around 150m (500ft) from the summit. Aged 21, I was too young to openly process the decisions I had made in that extreme environment. I used silence to help me find the peace I was seeking. Long walks and sitting alone in the garden

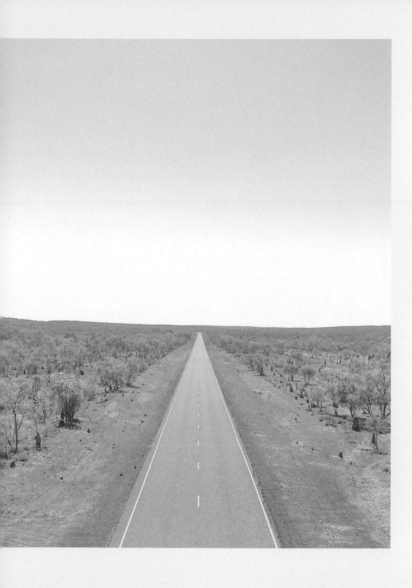

provided enough harmony to allow my mind to find comfort. Silence can be a meditative experience – not necessarily a focused period of yoga or meditation, but giving myself the opportunity to just be absorbed by my own thoughts, away from the stresses of life. Taking the time alone to silently reflect allowed me to evaluate my choices and come to terms with the outcome, move forward and subsequently complete my Seven Summits challenge by summiting Everest the following year.

The most influential period of silence I've experienced was not on an expedition but rather forcing myself to confront myself when writing my first book, *In Search of Sisu*. I opted to share an enormous amount of my life as a means to wholly portray the Seven Summits challenge I undertook, to potentially allow others to relate to my experiences and as a cathartic means of recovery from my mental health issues. Simply sitting down alone to write hour after hour was an emotionally intense period of silence that allowed a deeper level of self-awareness than I had previously experienced.

You've said that although ten minutes of mindfulness can be useful, there's something to be said for actually going on a journey. What do you know, based on your "extreme" experiences, that you wouldn't otherwise have known?

Taking that time, even just ten minutes a day, is beneficial. However, forcing yourself to cope with prolonged periods of isolation and reflection through a long journey is an entirely different kind of mindfulness. I have found that pushing myself out of my comfort zone, especially alone and especially over a sustained period of time, provides a means of emotional clarity I couldn't have experienced otherwise. The routine of cycling across monotonous landscapes, for instance, forces my mind to drift. With so few distractions, my brain is denied the opportunity to ignore the thoughts that come to the fore; it forces me to confront reality.

What benefits do you think increased silence could bring to all of us?

We are all capable of silence and self-reflection, but silence scares most people. Putting a mirror in front of your own failings and character flaws is a process that is emotionally demanding. Truly accepting your present with a whole understanding of your past is, however, the key to a new kind of freedom.

In your daily life at home, do you actively seek out silence? If so, where do you find it most easily?

The demands of commuting, jobs, people and technology in a daily working routine make silence harder to experience back at home. I have found that exercise and exploring in nature are the means by which I find time to process emotions and stress. The simplicity of taking time for myself, raising my pulse, experiencing an endorphin rush and being at ease with the outdoors is often all I need.

2

A HISTORY OF SILENCE

I never found anything as good
for the body as silence

Rabbi Simeon ben Gamliel

INTO THE DESERT
HERMITS AND THEIR LOVE OF SILENCE

Why have people through the ages sought to withdraw into silence, and how have these historic practices informed our understanding of silence today?

In the Christian tradition, the idea of withdrawing from the world into solitude and silence was first lived out in practice by the Desert Fathers and Mothers around the third century AD. Thousands of monks and nuns went to live in the desert, thereby laying the foundation for Christian monasticism as it still exists today. Many lived as hermits, whereas others banded together in small communities. Whether in complete solitude or companionship with others, they often practised extreme asceticism, by way of a strictly self-disciplined lifestyle devoid of any material or physical excesses.

Aside from fearing the complacency that comfort might bring, even more important to the hermits was the desire to lead a simple life that would allow more room for God's presence. Even today, silence is a key component of monastic life, and some monastic orders refer to themselves as "silent". Contrary to popular belief, however, none of them actually impose a vow of silence or practise complete silence. Most monasteries have specific times and places where speaking is prohibited unless absolutely necessary. Whether silent or speaking, all Christian monastic orders seek to refrain from idle talk, believing that it distracts from communication with God.

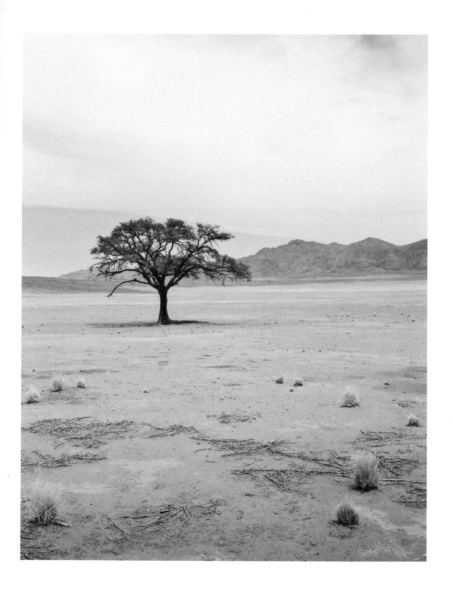

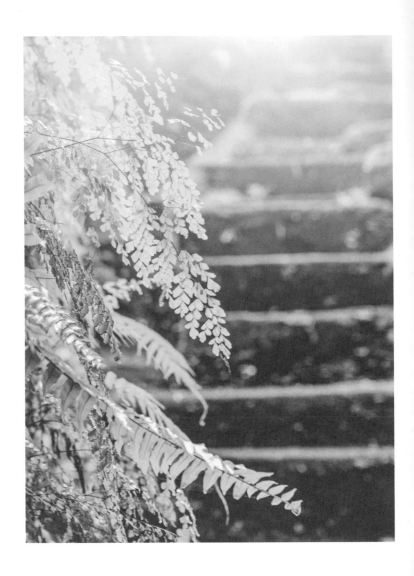

THE POWER OF QUIET
SILENCE IN ZEN BUDDHISM

Buddhist monasticism is one of the earliest forms of organized monasticism in the history of religion. Zen Buddhism, a school of Mahayana Buddhism, is varyingly defined as a practice, a philosophy and a way of life, the ultimate purpose of which is to achieve enlightenment. Enlightenment can be reached only through silence, and teachings can be understood only through silent meditation and contemplation. To the Zen practitioner, silence thus plays a key role in meditation as well as in life as a whole.

Zen Buddhism teaches that it is only through a quieting of one's mind that one can arrive at true insights; if there is noise (external noise as well as that of one's thoughts), it is not possible to see the true nature of things. The main forum for acquiring such insights is quiet meditation.

In Buddhism it is possible (although not required) to take a complete vow of silence.

THE SILENCE OF ETERNITY
THE SEARCH FOR GOD AND SELF

Every major religion and philosophy has an element of silence to it.

Judaism, traditionally perceived as focusing on words and books, teaches that God can reveal himself in silence and encourages an attentive, listening silence. In Islam, silence is viewed as a means of cultivating spirituality and nearness to Allah and as something integral to the faith.

In the religions of the Indian subcontinent, Hinduism, Buddhism and Jainism, there exists a concept of religious silence, called *mauna* or *mouna*, and the name for a sage is *muni*, literally meaning "silent one".

The ancient Greek philosopher Pythagoras (*c.*570–*c.*495BC) founded a school of philosophy whose disciples were characterized by their ascetic lifestyle and strictly observed vow of silence.

Over time silence has been admired, encouraged as a discipline, sought as something that could edify a person's mind and character, and often praised as a great virtue. It would seem that we used to have a less complicated relationship with silence than we do today. Interesting to ponder, then, how we have gone from that mindset to one that lauds constant action and subsequently sound.

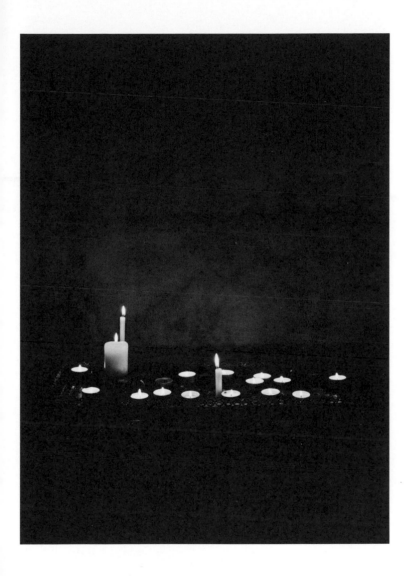

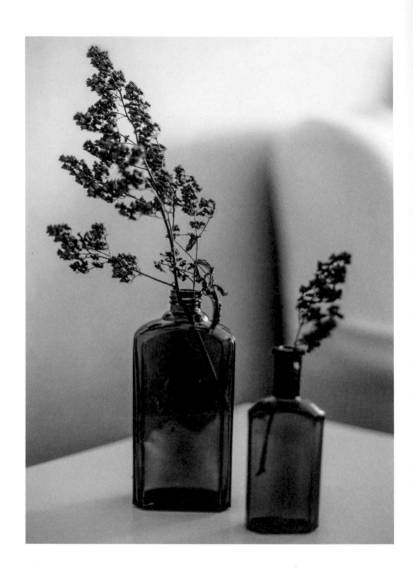

DON'T SPEAK
THE VOW OF SILENCE AS
STATEMENT AND TOOL

Just as silence in general can be perceived as alternately refreshing or difficult, silence between people is an equally complex beast. We see it in our language, where expressions such as "being silenced" make us think of repression, injustice and violence. There is a silence that diminishes, that is used as a means of exercising power over others; a silence that hinders life and growth. But in countering this negative silence, silence itself can become a powerful tool.

For instance, temporary vows of silence can be taken as a form of protest or to express a bold political statement. In the United States there is an annual Day of Silence, which is education organization GLSEN's day of action to spread awareness about the effects of the bullying and harassment of LGBTQ students. On this day, held in April each year since 1996, students take a day-long vow of silence to symbolically represent the silencing of LGBTQ students. Another example is the 30 November Vow of Silence for Free the Children, in which students in Canada are silent for 24 hours as a means of protesting against poverty and child labour.

Silent protests are used all over the world as a form of non-violent resistance, calling attention to injustice and corruption. As a mark of disapproval, silence can prove an effective agent of change.

WHEN WORDS ARE
NOT ENOUGH
A SHARED MOMENT OF SILENCE

When words fail us, we fall silent. Whether because of helplessness, grief or the impossibility of putting words to raging emotions, silence is sometimes our only recourse. This does not need to be a bad thing. Words have their uses and their time, but so does silence. Resorting to silence can be a sign of ultimate reverence or inexpressible sorrow. Natural disasters, genocide, tragedies, shocking acts of terrorism or simply remembering those fallen in battle – for a variety of reasons, most of us have observed a public minute (or several) of silence.

The first recorded instance of an official moment of silence to mark a person's death took place in Portugal on 13 February 1912, when the Portuguese Senate dedicated ten minutes of silence to a minister in the Brazilian government who had recently died. In the same year, large parts of the US kept a ceremonial silence to honour the dead of the USS *Maine* and the *Titanic*.

In the UK and across the Commonwealth, a two-minute silence is observed at 11am on Armistice Day (11 November) each year in remembrance of the sacrifices made by members of the armed forces and civilians in times of war.

In Israel, a moment of silence is held in memory of the victims of the Holocaust on Yom HaShoah ("Holocaust and Heroism Remembrance Day"), bringing the whole country to a dramatic standstill.

The practice of observing a moment's silence has become a global phenomenon, due at least partly to the fact that no single faith or philosophy can claim silence for itself. Silence can be used by anyone, anywhere, and as such it is a unique way for people of all faiths and none to engage in a shared ritual.

What Happens in Silence

Notes From a Visit to the Quakers

—

The Quakers, a historically Christian group of movements also known as The Religious Society of Friends, are characterized by freedom of thought and worship and the absence of authoritarian leadership. The liberty of each Quaker to freely interpret principles of Quakerism such as truth, justice, peace, integrity and simplicity means that practices vary greatly. One thing that binds Quakers together, however, is the regular habit of coming together in silence.

Curious to understand more about this practice, I contact the local Quaker community and am promptly invited to the next meeting.

I'm the only stranger this Sunday and the group welcomes me warmly. The meeting is due to start at 11am, and in the minutes leading up to it there is relaxed chatter. Then, without anyone taking the lead or saying anything, everybody suddenly grows quiet. The room we meet in is located in a basement and at first feels a little claustrophobic. Two small windows let in a little daylight, but we are still dependent on lamps. Chairs have been placed in a semi-circle. Aside from the occasional sound of someone walking by outside, it is quiet, and soon the only sound to be heard is that of other people in the room breathing.

Once we get going, the concerns I had beforehand – what if I sneeze or cough? Have forgotten to turn off my phone? Or worse, have to go to the bathroom? – start to fade. The atmosphere is far from tense, and despite sitting here with a group of complete strangers I soon find myself relaxing.

I hadn't made up my mind beforehand what to think about

during this hour, whether to pray, consciously meditate on something or just let my mind wander, but minute by minute the need for an agenda disappears. The initial oddness of the experience also wears off.

Some keep their eyes open, some shut. One woman has a warm little smile playing on her lips. There is the occasional sigh or yawn or sound of people shifting around in their chairs. I don't have a watch but am conscious of the wall clock behind me steadily ticking away.

If I didn't have at least a little experience of sitting motionless in silence, I suspect my mind would struggle to find a foothold in this "ocean of time" that opens up. After a while I'm quite sure that around half an hour has passed, but after that I lose my concept of time. It seems to flow of its own accord and I just drift with the current. Time no longer feels quantifiable but, curiously enough, I have also lost interest in keeping track of it.

Afterward it strikes me that this is perhaps the first time in my life that I have had a sense of actually *listening* to time as it passes. Time obviously flows whether I pay any attention to it or not, but enjoying this kind of prolonged silence seems to reveal its very movement: slow, steady, unhurried. Time is no longer running through my fingers, as it so often seems to do. It is ever arriving.

At one point, one of the women speaks – completely naturally and conversationally, as if she hadn't just broken a long silence. This, too, is part of Quaker custom. Those who feel moved to speak do so, while the others listen without commenting. The woman talks for a few minutes and when she is finished the silence resumes.

What I perceive as just a little while later (but I'm no longer sure), so simultaneously that it is as though a silent sign has passed between them, everyone suddenly stands up. I, too, scramble to my feet, a little late. We silently hold hands in the circle and exchange glances. I know that this signifies *thank you for sharing the silence with me*. It is a beautiful, strangely moving moment, and quite unlike anything I have experienced before.

After this, as naturally as anything, the group relaxes into chatter and several people eagerly begin sharing with me some things they think I ought to know. I ask a few follow-up questions, conscious of how slowly and quietly I am talking. The silence seems to cling to me still and it feels almost a little sacrilegious to speak, as if my words somehow risk polluting the room.

I'm struck by how naturally the group eases back into talking. It must have something to do with the practice of silence, I think; to them, being silent has lost its awkwardness and has become as natural as speaking.

How many people can claim to have a balance of silence and sound in their lives? Not many.

The Power of Collective Quiet
The small group I visit is in itself proof of the diversity that exists within the Quaker movement The silence, too, is perceived and used somewhat differently, but the one thing everybody seems to agree on is the great difference between communal and private silence.

Those I meet are more than happy to talk about the silence they practise but, unsurprisingly, the experience does not easily lend itself to being put into words. In between speaking they smile apologetically, interjecting phrases such as "It's hard to explain...", "How shall I describe it...?"

I think I understand. Aside from being just a peaceful practice, the Quaker silence is a meeting place with the Divine that shouldn't be deprived of its sacredness by the use of too many words. There is an expression in Swedish that roughly translates as "talking something to pieces" and I don't want to be guilty of that here, or of coaxing anyone to say more than they should. However, the practical impact that this silent hour has on their lives proves easier to approach and two members of the community were happy to share their thoughts on this:

It's difficult to explain the significance of the silence, except to say it means the world to me. I live alone, so there is no lack of silence at home if I want it. But this silence is very different. I'm one of the most active members of this community simply because I really need the silence! In it, I feel supported by the others. It makes a great difference to my mental health.

My times in silence at home are not at all like this. Sharing the silence makes all the difference somehow. Sure, I still get distracted. It's only natural, especially if there's a lot going on in my life. Engaging in this silence does get easier with time, but distractions will always be part of it to some degree. However, I always feel peaceful afterward. That's the interesting thing: it's always worth it. It has a lingering effect and infuses my life with calm.

For a 21st-century person, sitting in silence with a group of people for a whole hour is an irregular, fascinating and potentially frightening experience. It also feels rare and exclusive, like a gem. My own desire for silence meant I looked forward to it and wasn't disappointed, but that's not to say someone else wouldn't find it stressful.

But there is something here that intrigues me deeply. The Quakers themselves seem to experience silence as a unifying force, a means of building and strengthening community. Far from being a solitary pursuit, their silence edifies them as a group. And I, too, though just visiting, got a taste of the quite inexplicable sense of togetherness that emerges through sharing silence with other people.

Silence is a great equalizer. In silence, it is not possible to perform. Communal silence can act as an invitation to lay down our ego-driven agendas, our constant need to compete and outshine each other in order to "get ahead". With silence there is no getting ahead. Quite the opposite: it feels like an affirmation of our equal value and vulnerability as human beings. And I can't help wondering what untapped strength there is here, in this coming together in silence, that the world could benefit from accessing.

Silence is God's first language

St John of the Cross

JOYFUL NOISE
WHEN PEACE AND QUIET DON'T MEET

My visit to the Quakers led me to reflect on my own religious background. The church I grew up in was outwardly the very opposite of the Quakers. The Pentecostal movement, established in the early 20th century, is an emotionally expressive, loud denomination, marked by its adherence to freedom of worship. That freedom has inevitably meant noise. It is not uncommon for churchgoers to all pray aloud at the same time, or to shout approval in the middle of the message. The music is modern and amplified. Meetings, especially large ones, are usually relaxed, with people milling about.

Unsurprisingly, I can't recall there being any instances of silence at these meetings, either spontaneous or scheduled. It took me years to realize why I found this supposedly liberated environment so stressful. I now understand that my kind of personality needs silence in order to concentrate and be properly present.

Traditional churches place more emphasis on silence. To this day, the idea of seeking God in silence is worked out in the lives of men and women who choose to withdraw into convents, where the rhythm of daily life is marked out by alternating periods of togetherness and solitude, words and silence. Many churches also weave silence into the fabric of the service, often as recurring moments of quiet reflection.

This is partly why, despite words, music and the presence of other people, I tend to experience such church services as "silent" – simply because there is space for silence to be created within me.

What this has taught me is that we sometimes search high and low for reasons why a certain environment doesn't feel like a good fit for us, overlooking what might actually be a simple physiological explanation. Understanding how we as individuals are wired, how differently we experience the world, and what kind of environment we thrive in the most can go a long way toward increasing harmony in our lives.

SILENCE AND THE MODERN MIND
NATURE AS SANCTUARY

The desire to withdraw into silence has, of course, never been the prerogative of spiritual people alone. A growing and universal need for it has made itself felt since the Industrial Revolution. Here are several examples of thinkers who have helped shape our modern understanding of a world where the balance between nature and city, silence and noise has become crucially important.

Henry David Thoreau (1817–62)

An American naturalist, philosopher, poet and early environmentalist whose classic work *Walden* is an account of the two years he spent living alone in a log cabin in the woods by Walden Pond, Massachusetts. Thoreau sought the simple life that nature could provide and wrote extensively and often humorously about daily life as a voluntary hermit.

John Muir (1838–1914)

A Scottish-American naturalist and environmental philosopher also known as "John of the Mountains", Muir was an early pioneer of conservationism and is widely credited with having helped the preservation of America's national parks. His essays about adventures in the wild inspired generations of Americans to seek out nature for themselves. Muir's love of nature was influenced by his belief that the natural environment "came straight from the hand of God, uncorrupted by civilization and domestication";

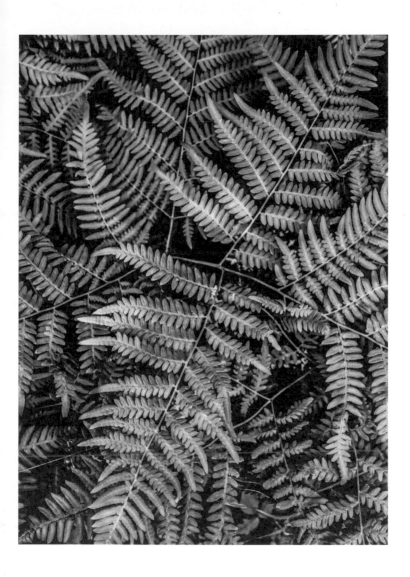

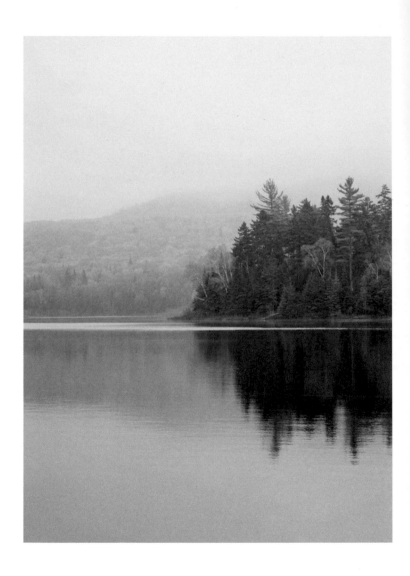

and he frequently praised "the wild" as being our true home, superior to civilization.

Annie Dillard (born 1945)

A modern-day American naturalist with the soul and pen of a poet, Dillard won the 1975 Pulitzer Prize for her *Pilgrim at Tinker Creek*, an account of a year spent in Virginia's Roanoke Valley. Her keen eye takes notes on nature in extreme and sometimes harrowing detail, all the while creating a deeply philosophical, soaring narrative of her sojourn in the wild.

Sara Maitland (born 1950)

Even more recently, this British author's *A Book of Silence* details her quest to make silence a key component of her life by retreating to live in the Scottish wilderness and spending long periods in complete silence. In so doing, she draws on a wide variety of sources of inspiration, from the Desert Fathers to modern-day explorers.

What these writers have in common is an extraordinary reverence for nature, shot through with a yearning for a time and a way of being that no longer exist. Without resorting to melancholy, their writing testifies to the fact that we are no longer completely at home in our natural state and need to be inspired to return there. Like silence, nature just *is* – sufficient unto itself.

3

NUMBING NOISE, SOOTHING SILENCE

All of humanity's problems stem from
one single thing: the inability to sit
quietly in a room alone

Blaise Pascal

NAUSEATING NOISE
THE INVISIBLE POLLUTANT

We live in an increasingly loud world. How does noise affect our health? And conversely, what are some of the ways in which silence impacts us?

The world we live in is louder than ever, and silence is increasingly difficult to come by. We're constantly filling our ears with music, TV, radio and podcasts, as well as involuntarily absorbing a multitude of sounds in our daily environment. In addition to the distractions these sounds cause, constantly living with noise may be negatively affecting our health. Perhaps it is no coincidence that the word *noise* derives from *nausea*.

"Some day people will be incessantly fighting noise the same way we have fought cholera and plague," predicted German physician and microbiologist Robert Koch as early as the 1800s. He was proved right (if he hadn't been before) in 2011 when a World Health Organization report referred to noise pollution as a "modern plague", concluding that "there is overwhelming evidence that exposure to environmental noise has adverse effects on the health of the population". The study calculated that the 340 million residents of Western Europe annually lost a million years of healthy life because of noise.

WHY NOISE IS MAKING US SICK
SOUND VS STRESS

Sound waves reach the brain as electrical signals via the ear. The body reacts to these signals even during sleep. Noise stimulates the nervous system and has a strong physical effect on our brains, raising the levels of stress hormones. In response to loud noise, the amygdala, a part of the brain associated with memory and emotion, releases higher levels of the stress hormone cortisol. If you live in a consistently noisy environment, you are therefore likely to experience chronically elevated levels of stress hormones. This increases the risk of hypertension, which in turn has been connected to many other cardiovascular and cerebrovascular diseases such as heart attacks and strokes.

As long ago as 1859, British nurse and social reformer Florence Nightingale wrote, "Unnecessary noise is the most cruel absence of care that can be inflicted on sick or well." She argued that careless clatter as well as needless chatter could prove harmful for recovering patients, and that good care, by contrast, was quiet.

Without even including the hearing damage that long-term exposure to loud noise may result in, we have a big problem on our hands.

Noise is one of the biggest pollutants in our cities, but – despite being linked to an increased risk of early death –

the issue is often overlooked. The rather interesting reason for this is that we are good at adapting to background noise – perhaps too good. But even if we subconsciously tune out the unwanted noise until it doesn't bother us anymore, it still affects us. A good example of this is demonstrated by a study published in 2002 in *Psychological Science*, examining the effects that the relocation of Munich's airport had on local children's health and cognition. The study showed that children who are exposed to noise develop a response mechanism that allows them to ignore it. But curiously, this is not limited to potentially harmful noise – it also includes sounds they should be paying attention to, such as speech. Studies have also concluded that children whose homes or schools are located near airplane flight paths, railways or highways have lower reading scores and are slower in their development of cognitive and language skills.

Noise pollution harms performance at work and at school. It can also be the cause of decreased motivation and an increase in errors. The cognitive functions that are most strongly affected by noise are reading attention, memory and problem solving.

CAN YOU HEAR ME?

The following are examples of typical decibel levels of sounds we may all experience in the course of our lives.

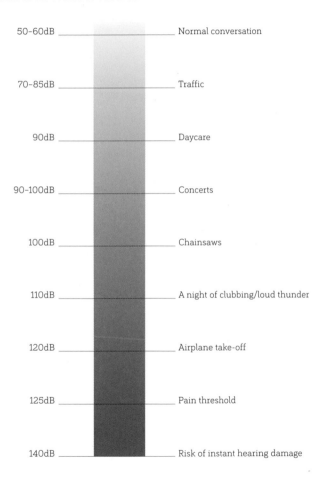

50–60dB	Normal conversation
70–85dB	Traffic
90dB	Daycare
90–100dB	Concerts
100dB	Chainsaws
110dB	A night of clubbing/loud thunder
120dB	Airplane take-off
125dB	Pain threshold
140dB	Risk of instant hearing damage

HEADPHONES AND
HEARING LOSS
AN UNCOMFORTABLE TRUTH

Can't hear anything else when you listen to music through headphones? Then the volume is too high. Most MP3 players produce sounds up to 120dB. At that level, hearing loss can occur after only about an hour and 15 minutes.

A 2011 study published in the *Journal of the American Medical Association* showed that one in five teens experience some form of hearing loss, an increase of 30 per cent over 20 years. Many believe this escalation is due to the increased use of headphones. Experts agree that the problem is twofold: our hearing is affected by both the volume and the length of exposure to sound. In other words, listening through headphones or earbuds at a moderate volume can also damage hearing over time. Considering how dependent we have become on tuning out the world around us with the help of headphones, this is bad news. So what should we do?

When using headphones, a good rule of thumb is "60/60": don't exceed 60 per cent of your music player's maximum volume and use your headphones for at most 60 minutes per day. Other recommendations are to use over-the-ear headphones rather than in-ear ones, and to choose the noise-cancelling kind: they will allow you to hear music at lower volumes, making you less likely to crank it up.

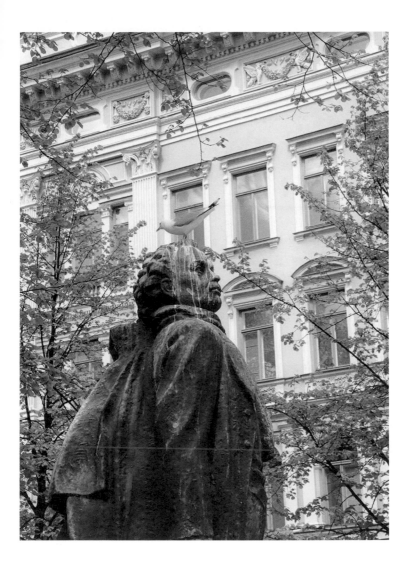

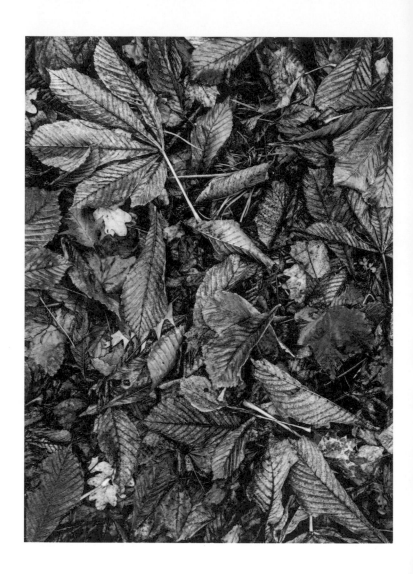

THE ANTIDOTE
HOW SILENCE GROWS YOUR BRAIN

Just as too much noise can cause stress, tension and possibly illness, research has shown that silence has the opposite effect. A 2006 study published in the journal *Heart* found that two minutes of silence were more relaxing than listening to "relaxing" music, based on changes in blood pressure and blood circulation in the brain.

In our everyday lives, sensory input comes at us from all directions. When we get away from these sonic disruptions, our brain's capacity for attention gets the opportunity to restore itself. A 2013 study on mice, published in the journal *Brain, Structure, and Function*, involved comparing the effects of ambient noise, white noise, pup calls and silence on the rodents' brains. Although the researchers intended to use silence only as a control in the study, they found that two hours of silence daily led to the development of new cells in the hippocampus, the brain region involved in memory formation.

As it turns out, an *absence* of input proved to have more impact than any actual input.

DEFAULTING TO SILENCE
THE BENEFITS OF A WANDERING MIND

Our brains have something that researchers call the default mode network. It is active when our brains rest from obvious tasks, when we engage in, for example, daydreaming, meditating, fantasizing about the future or just letting our minds wander. The default mode is also involved when we engage in self-reflection.

In order to return to its default mode, the brain needs times of idleness when it doesn't have to react to any demanding external stimuli. Silence is obviously a very efficient way of achieving this.

When not distracted by noise or goal-orientated tasks, the brain allows us to tap into our inner thoughts, emotions, memories and ideas. The default mode helps us make sense of our experiences, but also to empathize with others and reflect on our own mental and emotional states. All deep and creative thinking takes place in the default mode.

It is not hard to imagine the mental fatigue that follows when the brain is consistently kept from reaching this restorative state. Although always active in some way, the brain differentiates sharply between different kinds of activity. It is therefore not an exaggeration to say that the brain needs periods of silence in order to function properly.

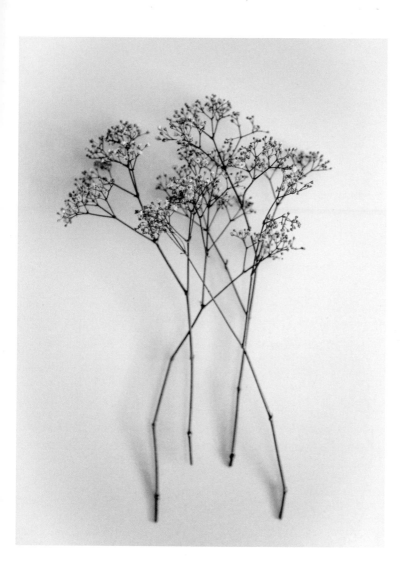

4

A SILENT MIND

Silence is the mother of truth

Benjamin Disraeli

SILENCE AVOIDANCE
HOW FAR WOULD YOU GO?

Silence is often perceived as a negative phenomenon, something that causes our anxiety levels to soar. Why is this and what can we do to make friends with it?

A study reported in 2014 in the journal *Science* found that many people chose to self-administer an electric shock rather than sit quietly in a room alone with their thoughts.

For the experiment, researchers brought people into their lab and asked them to sit alone in an empty room. Every kind of stimulus – mobile phones, watches, music players and so on – was taken away. The researchers pointed out a nearby button, which, when pressed, would give the participant an electric shock.

Each participant was asked to press the button once, to rate the unpleasantness of the shock and then to say whether they would pay money not to be shocked again. The participants said the shock was unpleasant enough that they would pay to avoid it.

After they had been introduced to the shock button, the participants were asked to sit alone in the room and entertain themselves with their own thoughts for 10 to 20 minutes. There were only two rules: they weren't allowed to get out of their chair and they couldn't fall asleep. And should they like to receive another electric shock, the button was there for them to push.

Despite having already said they would pay money to avoid being shocked again, about 70 per cent of the men and 25 per cent of the women chose to shock themselves during that short interval, instead of sitting idly with their own thoughts. Some did it multiple times.

The study concluded that, when faced with the sheer unpleasantness of being alone with their thoughts, "most people prefer doing something to nothing, even if that something is negative".

Silence is the sleep that nourishes wisdom

Francis Bacon

Silence – Awkward and Scary or Revelatory and Inspiring?

In order to understand why so many of us view silence as something to be avoided at all costs, I turn to psychologist Dr Olga Lehmann, who has researched and published extensively on silence and its role in psychotherapy as well as in other contexts, such as the relationship between art and silence, and silence in music. She has developed a theory about silence phenomena, in other words all the experiences associated with the word "silence".

Why do you think we often find silence difficult or frightening?

Far from being empty, silence is introspective space. A tension arises in this silent space, and we have to dare to go into it, into this field of tension. It takes courage, because we don't know how to handle this and how to sustain ourselves in silence. We're not used to it anymore.

You would like us to invite more silence into our lives. Why?

Silence is a space for emotional experiences. My experience and my research show that a tremendous amount of processes occur in this space.

Psychology tends to rely heavily on words to articulate feelings and experiences. In your view, can silence accomplish different and perhaps better results?

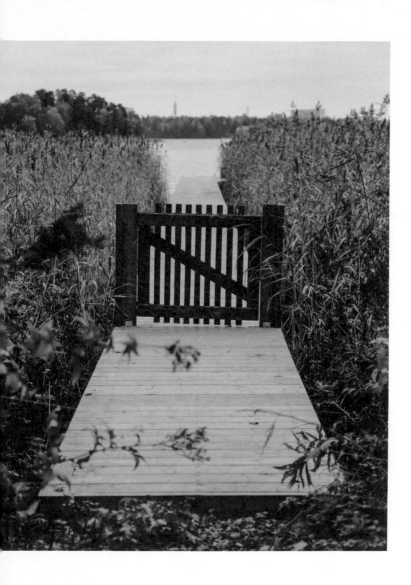

Psychologists like to do interviews and surveys, and to talk. But everyone knows how hard it can be to put words to certain feelings and that we struggle to explain some of our deepest life experiences in words. I consider this when I teach, often beginning my classes with a time of silence that students can later reflect on. I find silence to be a great catalyst for emotions.

What about those unpleasant feelings, how should we approach them?

Silence might make you afraid. But don't forget it can still give you something, even when you find it awkward. Silence often emphasizes our sense of uncertainty, but this is part of life and nothing to be afraid of. I would encourage everyone to be less afraid of entering into silence.

Another thing you have uncovered in your research is that our emotional life is more complex than was previously thought. Could you elaborate?

Some psychological theories maintain that we have only one main feeling at a time, but my investigations of silence show that we have several emotions in parallel. Our mind is like a small community, or like a theatre with many characters on stage simultaneously. And these characters can speak with conflicting voices and opinions. For example, my students who had to deal with silence were both frustrated and satisfied at the same time. Don't hesitate to embrace the complexity inherent in silence: that silence can be several things at once.

What would you say are some of the practical ways in which silence can improve our lives?

Your own silence can make it easier for you to listen to others. It can also be used to listen to your own inner voice. Silence gives us the opportunity to create depth in our relationships, whether with other people, with nature or with God. It also gives us an opportunity to deepen our relationship with ourselves. I also believe silence can result in better decision-making, both in one's own life and in business, simply because silence gives us more room for reflection. Not least of all, silence is a great facilitator of experiences that I call "poetic instants", a notion coined by my favourite poet, Mexican Nobel laureate Octavio Paz. Poetic instants are moments in our everyday life that may be filled with aesthetic experiences, nature appreciation or perhaps love.

Do you have any encouraging words for those of us who are doubtful about even finding silence in the first place?

Silence is everywhere – we just need to pay attention to it. Try to identify the silence when you come across it in your daily life. Try to discern if you are comfortable with it, or if it pains you. And above all: use the silence to become more attentive.

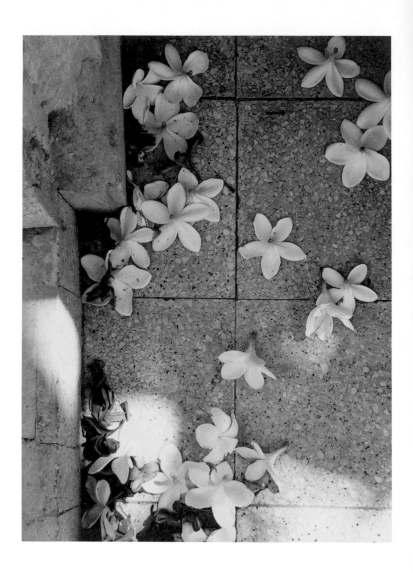

SILENT TOGETHER
SILENCE IN RELATIONSHIPS

Silence between two people who are close can be beautifully companionable. There is a deep peace in knowing you are loved and accepted. Words become superfluous; sometimes they even get in the way. Sharing silences like these with the man I love, or as a child sitting quietly in my mother's arms, is the closest I've experienced being to another person.

"You could cut the silence with a knife" – this expression can also hold true for that close relationship. A silence that is choking with unspoken – and unspeakable – words, a silence marking the gulf that has opened up between two people. Such silences are oppressive and cry out to be broken.

Most of us know the painful silence that results from a complete breakdown in communication. When words have been spoken but to no avail, silence sometimes becomes our only recourse. We think of reaching out, of calling or writing, but keep coming back to the futility of it. Far from being mute, this uncomfortable silence speaks volumes.

There is nothing conclusive to say about silence in relationships, except to acknowledge its dual role. Silence can be comforting, but it can also act as an alarm clock. Whichever of these is the case, simply paying attention to the silence when it occurs is key to being able to use it well.

FIGHTING THE NOISE
WHEN TECHNOLOGY COMES
BETWEEN US

When it comes to simultaneously removing fruitful silence – the kind that gives rise to great conversations – and promoting the kind that causes people to drift apart, constant connectedness has become public enemy number one.

In 2015, a study at Brigham Young University in Utah coined the term *technoference* to describe the harmful effect that intrusions and interferences by technology devices have on romantic relationships, leading to feelings of rejection and outright depression. Referencing the study, the journal *Psychology Today* concluded that whereas the main disputes for couples used to be about sex, money and childrearing, smartphone usage is skyrocketing up the list.

When Finnish newspaper *Helsingin Sanomat* conducted a survey in 2019 for the purpose of finding out what constant smartphone usage does to romantic relationships, they weren't expecting to find what the paper referred to as a "unanimous cry for help" rising from the hundreds of answers received. Respondents complained about partners being constantly online and always ready to have a real-life conversation interrupted, to the point where things happening on the phone took precedence over the person actually present in the room. Most confessed to being equally part of the problem. Even when faced with the dramatic deterioration of the relationship, this bad habit has proved notoriously hard to break.

This is a pandemic and it is serious. Functioning, healthy relationships form the bedrock of our physical and mental wellbeing. The future of those relationships, our quality of life, mental health and family cohesiveness may depend on us clearing the space necessary for silence to occur. Giving our partner our full attention and the equivalent of a blank page to write on is rapidly becoming the most romantic gesture imaginable.

—

Losing My Silence

Panic Attacks and the "S" Word

—

It is late at night. Very late, in fact, but I can't sleep. After postponing going to bed for as long as possible, I now lie here wishing I was someone else, somewhere else. I feel as if I'm about to crawl out of my skin. My pulse is rapid and I'm breaking out in a cold sweat, as waves of something I can't name wash over me with renewed force every few minutes. I want to phone somebody just to hear their voice, as a reminder of life still going on in places where normal people go to bed without fearing for their sanity. But I don't. I wouldn't know what to say.

A panic attack. That's what I was having, and continued to have every night for a period of several months. It was only when the feelings returned some years later that I was able to put a name to this harrowing experience. By that time I also knew that not only was I not going insane, I was far from alone in feeling the way I did.

Panic attacks can manifest in different ways and be triggered by many different situations. It took me a long time to connect that first period of attacks with the breakup I had recently gone through. It didn't make any sense – I felt relief at the relationship ending, after all. I wasn't used to the solitude but had always enjoyed spending time by myself, so what was the problem?

Eventually, things just settled and falling asleep became easier. I was glad to return to normal and didn't spend any more time dwelling on my experiences.

When the sensations returned, years later, I was at first as mystified as before. My father had died ten months earlier, while my husband and I were living abroad. We spent some time at home after his passing and then flew back to our very busy life elsewhere. It was only when we returned for good the next year that my panic attacks resurfaced and I slowly began to realize that not only had I postponed the grieving process, but that the very bedrock of my life had been shaken when my father died. The first time around, the trigger had been something similar: not an equally seismic shift, but a shaking of my world nevertheless.

The thing I hated most about my panic attacks was the sudden fear of silence. I had always loved solitude and enjoyed quiet. Now they were being taken away from me, and for a long time I felt like a tightly wound string – pluck at it just a little and it will break. Constantly needing people and sounds around just in order to function

normally is not a sustainable lifestyle and there were times when I despaired about my future. There was suddenly no way for me to truly relax, and living for longer periods of time with such high levels of stress is exhausting. Worse still, putting words to my feelings was proving difficult, and I felt myself silenced in the midst of all the noise.

Gift or Curse?

From reading testimonies by other panic attack sufferers I've learned that a commonly shared experience at the onset of an attack is the fear that one's whole self may be disintegrating. In that frightening place, silence can feel very dangerous. The very thing that is necessary for healthy introspection becomes something to shun at all costs. Silence is a blank sheet, after all, and when thoughts become scary, silence is perceived as the thing that will push us over the edge.

I got well in the end. It was a gradual process, without a clear turning point or reason. I wish I had a panacea that would instantly cure all forms of panic attack, but the only thing I know for sure happened was that I began to talk about how I felt. By breaking the silence, as it were, I got silence back again. Since I lost it for a time, I don't think I shall ever stop being grateful for the simple pleasure of feeling good in the absence of sound.

Do I consider myself cured of panic attacks? Not necessarily. When big changes occur in my life I know to be on the lookout for tremors under the surface of my mind, and to exercise generous self-love. For me that means eating and sleeping well, moving my body, getting fresh air and feeding my mind with uplifting things. And, I'm very pleased to say, spending time by myself in silence.

Silence is a source of Great Strength

Lao Tzu

RETREATING FROM IT ALL
GOING AWAY TO BE SILENT

If you enjoy silence and you long to explore it some more, or you are just feeling curious about it, there are some interesting options to consider.

One alternative to a full-on hermit existence is to go on a retreat for a few days. They are offered in a variety of environments, at varying lengths and may be centred on a creed or meditation technique.

The basic premise of a retreat is to spend some time outside normal life, in a different place and with a different daily rhythm. Of necessity, a certain asceticism is also part of the package: after all, what would be the point of retreating if everything we sought to take a break from were coming with us? Many retreats impose strict rules on internet usage, for instance, or regulate the amount of speaking that goes on.

retreat (ri'tri:t) *n.* **1** an act or process of withdrawing, especially from what is difficult, dangerous or disagreeable **2** a place of privacy or safety **3** a period of group withdrawal for prayer, meditation, study or instruction

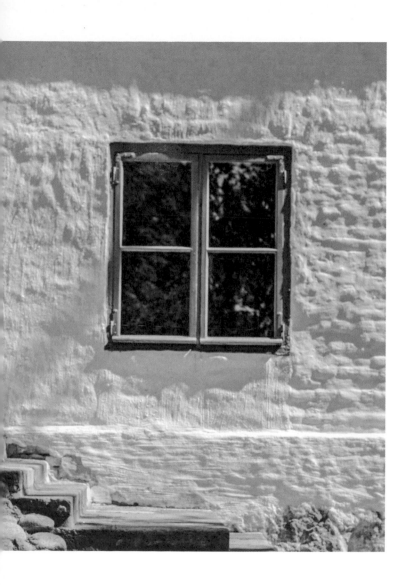

Face to Face with Silence – The Challenge of Introspection

To find out more about retreating from it all, I spoke to journalist Emelie Wikblad, who spent a few days on a silent retreat and wrote an article about the experience that she titled "Silence is the reward – and the challenge". The retreat incorporated different Christian monastic traditions, and shared times of coming together to sing or meditate were part of the daily rhythm.

You write how, at the start of the retreat, nobody cared to say much even while speaking was still allowed. You ended up spending several days with these people, in complete silence – did that feel odd?

Not really. I suppose people who seek out a silent retreat do so out of a longing to refrain from speaking and come mentally prepared for that. I myself am an introvert and find small talk to be hard work sometimes; to take a break from having to obey these social conventions was a relief. Silence doesn't place any demands on us. It was refreshing, not being called upon to perform socially.

Without mobile phones, TV and speaking to other people, it's easy to assume that time passes very slowly. Did it?

The whole retreat followed a set rhythm and we were told beforehand what we'd be doing. There was a list of key times on the wall, but we never had to keep track of time for ourselves. A bell would ring five minutes before each scheduled activity, for instance a time of meditation. Having someone else manage your time is liberating and I did experience that time began to flow differently. Also, not having anything you "have" to do and no phone to check means that normal everyday things are allowed to take more time. I noticed we all gradually began moving more slowly, taking longer to eat, that sort of thing. Actually being in the present became a lot easier.

The only occasion when I felt time was passing slowly was in the hour or so before going to bed. I spent this time reading, which actually made me realize how little reading I'd done lately – there is always an interesting film or TV series that tends to win out. It made me resolve to spend more time reading. But on the whole, that time slot felt a little too quiet.

What was most difficult?

Doing so much introspection. After a few days I really couldn't find anything new to meditate or reflect on, I felt pretty done. As a result, I was a bit restless and fidgety on the last day, and felt ready to return to my normal life.

What did you take away from this experience and who would you recommend it for?

Afterward I felt calmer and more grounded. I also had a sense of renewed gratitude for those things we usually take for granted, like social media or easy access to different things. Like most people, I'm very used to being constantly connected and it was great to take a break from that. For that reason I would recommend a retreat for anyone. Having said that, I'm comfortable with silence and don't find it oppressive. Someone who isn't used to it at all may want to start small. There are silent retreats as long as ten days or more, but I'm certain that's something you need to work your way up to!

Would you do it again, for instance during a stressful period?

I would. But I think I'd try something a bit more active. For instance, there are outdoor retreats where you go hiking together in silence. For me personally, being active helps me think and calm down a lot easier than just sitting still in one spot. Challenging yourself is always good, but there is also the freedom to let the kind of personality you have inform your choice of retreat.

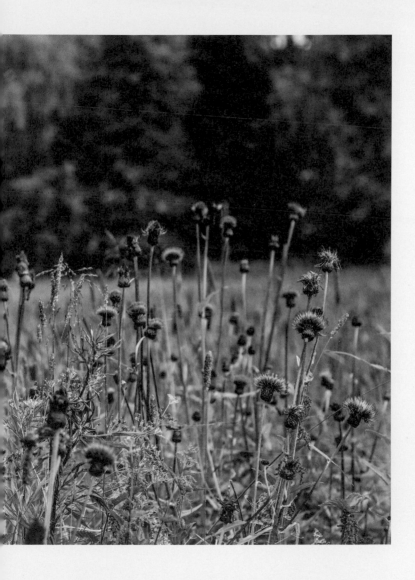

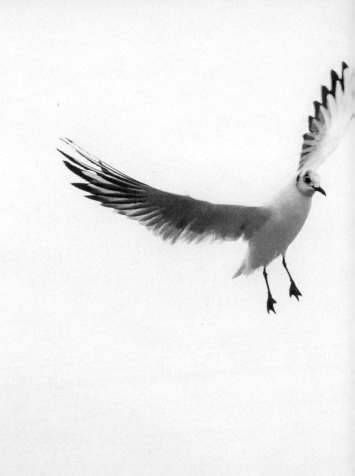

5

FINDING SILENCE

In order to see birds it is necessary to
become a part of the silence

Robert Lynd

THE HOME OF SILENCE
NATURE WORKING ITS MAGIC

Where do we go in search of silence? Nature is an obvious choice, but thankfully the city, too, offers silent spaces and activities. The focus of this chapter is on whether or not it is possible to accommodate our need for silence even in a bustling metropolis.

When it comes to silence, there is one environment above all that acts as a speed dial of connection – nature.

Although not strictly silent, nature sounds don't have the same effect on us as other types of noise. (Have you ever heard anyone complaining about birdsong being stressful?) Deserts, wilderness and seas offer the most sublime of solitudes, and many who venture there alone speak of a gradually growing, uncanny sense of merging with nature and becoming one with the landscape. But even if we can't have nature all to ourselves (or would even wish to), it is still the most restorative environment available to us.

It is, of course, no secret that nature is extremely good for us in all kinds of ways. It is, after all, our natural habitat. Unfortunately, it can be hard to come by. Even more important, then, to consciously make whatever is available a part of our lives. And even very little is better than nothing. Research shows that just looking at a picture of nature can give us an energy boost. (City vistas have no such effect.)

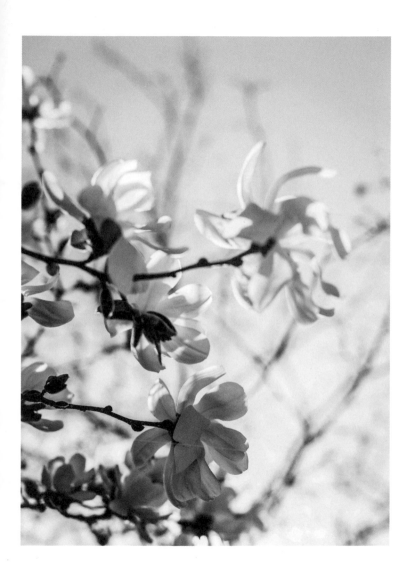

Pictures, green indoor plants and nature documentaries on television may seem like a poor substitute for the real thing, but they will still add rather than subtract something from your life.

Making the most of nature is obviously optimal, if we can. But even those of us with relatively easy access to green cathedrals may well not take full advantage of them. It takes a little effort, after all. If you're in doubt of its worth, however, why not try replacing 15 minutes of hunched-over scrolling with a stroll in a nearby park, and see for yourself if it makes a difference?

Spending time in nature by watching a sunset, gazing at the sea or a mountain, sitting in a park, escaping to the countryside or a nature retreat, or even just a few minutes staring out the window provides us with an opportunity to rest, reflect and become restored.

This points to another role that nature plays in our lives: contributing to overcoming mental fatigue and improving our ability to focus our mind and direct our attention. To get you inspired to get up and out, here are just a few of nature's many benefits.

Brain Gym – Nature Improves Memory and Concentration
In one study, University of Michigan students were given a small memory test before being divided into two groups. One group took a walk around an arboretum, the other down a city street. When the participants returned and retook the test, those who had walked among trees did almost 20 per cent better than they had the first time. Those who had taken in city sights instead saw no consistent improvement in their memory.

The effect nature has on our attention span is so strong that it may help children with ADHD, who have been shown to concentrate better after just 20 minutes in a park.

Nature Therapy – A Balm for the Stressed-out
Another study found that students sent into the forest for two nights had lower levels of cortisol – a hormone often used as a marker for stress – than those who spent corresponding time in the city. A different experiment found a decrease in both heart rate and levels of cortisol in subjects in the forest when compared with those in the city. Among office workers, even a view of nature from the window is associated with lower stress and higher job satisfaction.

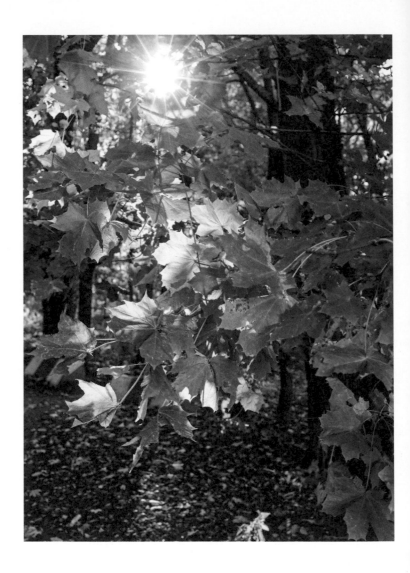

The Doctor Outside – Nature Can Heal Both Body and Mind

Anxiety, depression and other mental health issues may all be eased by some time in the great outdoors, especially when that's combined with exercise. One study found that there was a strong connection between walks in the forest and decreased levels of anxiety and bad moods; another found that outdoor walks could be "useful as a supplement to existing treatments" for major depressive disorders.

Spending time in nature may also help keep your immune system in check. In one study, elderly patients sent on a week-long trip into the forest showed reduced signs of inflammation. In another, students who spent time in the forest had lower levels of inflammation than a group who spent that time in the city. There is also evidence to suggest that nature provides a general boost to the immune system, helping your body fight off colds, flus and other infections.

All these benefits (and more) come in addition to the benefits of silence alone. So whether it's an activity of some sort or just taking it easy in a deckchair, time spent outside will have a positive impact on us. Making the most of the silence nature provides is, however, dependent on us actually leaving our headphones and the gadgets attached to them at home.

Silence Tourism – Making Silence and Nature Priorities When You Go Away

For those desperate to get away from it all, there is always the opportunity to seek out silence in remote places. High-end spa holidays in exotic locations or adventure tourism at high altitudes are all well and good, but finding silence doesn't necessarily require a thick wallet. Nature tourism, with hiking, fishing and camping on the agenda, is available in most countries. And for a restful staycation you may rent a cabin in a remote area, seek out a silent retreat in beautiful surroundings or spend a cosy weekend in a sleepy town – with silence first on the agenda, you may be surprised at the breadth of affordable options available.

I go to nature to be soothed and healed,
and to have my senses put in order

John Burroughs

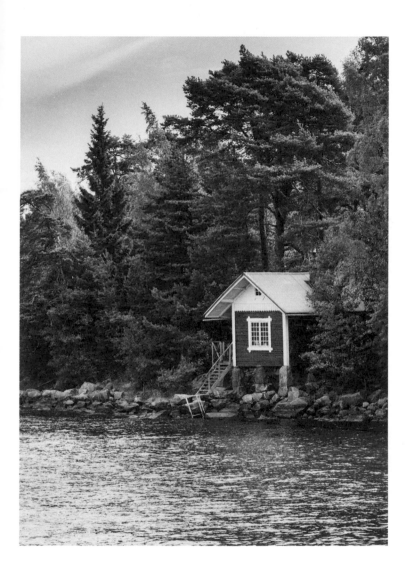

Silence on the High Seas – Sailing to the End of the World

Someone who knows a lot about the contrast between urban noise and Earth's most silent corners is Milo Dahlmann, the first Swedish woman to sail alone across the Atlantic. Ten years later, in 2009–11, in her boat *Artemisia II,* she fulfilled a life-long dream by sailing to Antarctica. Dahlmann has spent long stretches of time in some of the remotest waters on Earth and has written two books about her adventures.

You have spent months by yourself out at sea. Would you describe that loneliness as silent?

Yes and no. Compared with urban everyday life it is fantastically silent. There are lots of sounds, of course: the wind, birds, dolphins, the boat breaking through the waves...The inner silence, however, is amazing. You aren't constantly interrupted by other things vying for your attention. You get to actually finish a thought – or not think at all. You can rest your brain, allow yourself simply to meld with your environment until you feel part of it.

You write very honestly about how you sometimes experienced doubts and fears. Do you think people tend to shun silence precisely to avoid that?

When I'm out lecturing I often meet people who say, "I wouldn't dare to be alone even for a single day!" When I ask what it is that scares them, they will often say things

like "People wouldn't be able to reach me, what if something happened?" or "Without noise around me I'd be afraid the whole time."

Underneath these arguments is the fear of facing yourself. In order to know who we really are we have to dare to be alone with ourselves for a longer period of time, without access to phones, computers and TV. We need enough time to access what's behind the shell. This scares most people. But I am absolutely convinced that every single person in the world would benefit from it. Many people have completely lost sight of what is of lasting value in life. This makes us feel less than great, and we keep a lid on that by constantly keeping the focus away from ourselves. This actually causes our thinking to deteriorate. I do think people in general avoid silence to avoid having to feel.

You've shared how overwhelmed you were by the flow of input when you returned home, as your brain had to readjust to sorting through impressions rather than focusing on everything. Did you feel that living so intensely in the moment created a silence within you?

Absolutely. When we are away from all the regular impressions, I think our brains revert to their normal state. And normal is to see, feel and reflect on what is happening here and now. I would really prefer to be doing this all the time. But I had to shut down my alertness when I got home, purely to survive; our brains can't cope with being that open all the time.

Just over a year ago my partner and I and our cat moved to an island. And it didn't take long for my brain to start functioning somewhat similarly to when I was sailing long distances. Here we have no street lamps, no big roads, no airplanes flying over. I can hear the neighbour's rooster crowing and horses neighing. I can stop what I'm doing just to enjoy the sight of a deer passing by.

I do also have to go into the city and work for a living. And I'm really aware that all the noises, especially loud ones, affect me more negatively now than they used to. I take this as a positive sign!

What role do you think nature plays in our peace of mind?

The greatest role of all. We are part of nature and without it we cannot survive. If we cut out nature from our lives, we cut out our humanity at the same time.

In the world as a whole, it would seem that both internal and external silence is becoming rare. What do you think about that?

It frightens me. Without silence – internal as well as external – we can't think properly anymore. Our brains become unable to focus and think in long-term perspectives. Ultimately, we lose the ability to envision the consequences of our actions and decisions.

SILENCE AND THE CITY
IN SEARCH OF URBAN SANCTUARIES

Silent spaces in the city are notoriously hard to come by, but they do exist. Here are five examples.

1. Parks

An obvious one, you might think. But whereas most of us have an internal map of where the parks around us are, we tend to register the large ones and miss the small. Chances are that even the neighbourhood where your office is located has a small park tucked away somewhere. Smaller areas "left over" in city planning are often turned into park-like areas. See whether you can locate these in your residential or working area.

2. Quiet streets

We are creatures of habit and this also applies to the route we take to work. Make a point of getting to know your neighbourhood better. Every area has busier and quieter streets, and finding the latter may be just a small exploration away. Even in areas with a high density of people you can find surprisingly quiet urban backwaters. One-way streets are also always worth checking out for that reason.

3. Public buildings

Museums, public libraries, churches and chapels, even sections of airports and train stations can provide easy access to a time of silence.

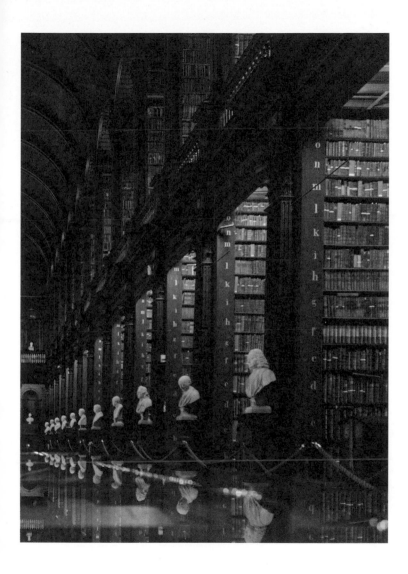

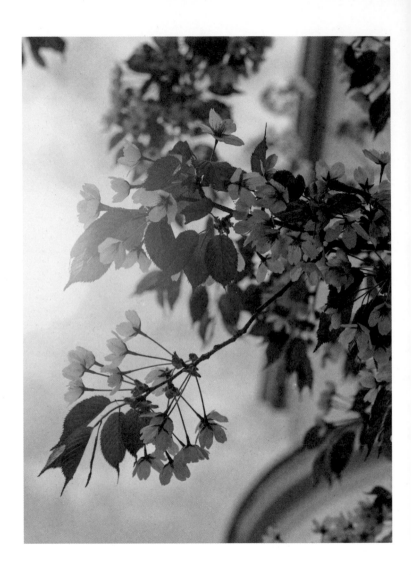

4. Cafés

This one might come as a surprise, but not all cafés are created equal. Especially in large cities it's not hard to come by places that aren't all that well frequented. It could be because the coffee is awful, but chances are they're simply located a little bit off the beaten track.

Another thing to investigate is that not all cafés play music. In fact, some have a policy never to do so. That won't necessarily mean they're quiet, but at least you've eliminated one major noise factor.

5. Botanical gardens

Most large cities have at least one botanical garden, and entrance to them is often free. The combination of silence and nature enjoyment that these green havens offer can prove the perfect antidote to a stressful day.

Building Quiet – An Architect's Thoughts on Silence

Looking at the structure of a city and the preconditions on which it is built – to act as a centre of commerce and entertainment that pulls people together – does silence get any room at all? Architect and writer Pirkko-Liisa Schulman is a graduate of the Helsinki University of Technology (now Aalto University) and Yale University. She has lectured, worked and published internationally and is also an architectural historian with experience of restoration projects. She tells me her views on:

Building silence

Considering different aspects of soundproofing is just part of the equation when it comes to constructing silent spaces. The surrounding environment with its buildings and traffic also needs to be taken into account. Even the climate, and phenomena such as wind tunnels, play a part in how silent a space can become. This is why city planning is so important. Somebody needs to have the bigger picture of the urban landscape that will emerge over time.

I would argue that when it comes to creating a peaceful environment, visual factors are just as important as noise reduction. Identical blocks of flats can be very depressing, but on the other hand, when every single building in your neighbourhood looks unique, it is difficult to find any harmony or construct a meaningful whole out of what you see. The environment becomes, in a manner of speaking, loud.

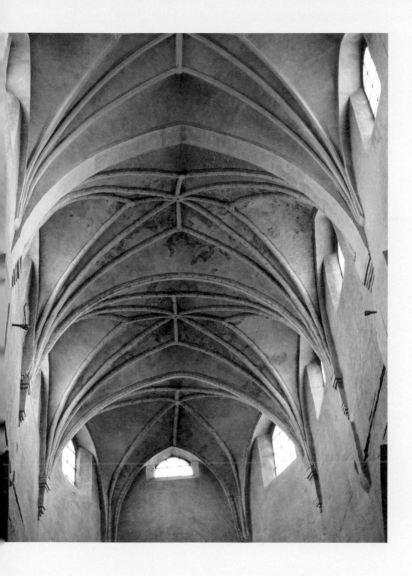

We architects are often blamed for just building white, white, white and favouring a very muted palette, but bold colours can be tricky. We don't all feel the same about them and this is why striving to achieve harmony is paramount in public spaces. I remember once sitting in a hospital waiting room, counting at least 20 colours around me! It was a very loud environment that just added to my anxiety.

Noise levels in the city

Traffic keeps increasing and there is always construction or repairs going on somewhere. We are hopefully past the age when everything – sometimes including beautiful old buildings – had to make way for the car. Still, we have a long way to go in making cities better environments to dwell in.

Something I notice a lot is the increase in sound from digital outdoor screens. Marketing used to be limited to shop windows and a few designated places; now it's ubiquitous. Walking through a shopping centre, you are assaulted by sounds and video from every side. This is unnecessarily distracting and could easily be regulated to create a quieter inner-city environment.

Visual noise

As a visual person, I'm always noticing things in the cityscape that are out of place or disharmonious. I wish we could declutter our cities, but they are dynamic and ever evolving.

With all the screens in our lives, the increase in moving images everywhere concerns me. It's really hard to avoid looking at them, which is, of course, the whole point. But they, too, are a form of noise pollution: creating environments that are restless and stressful, as well as potentially being a traffic hazard.

Silent spaces in the city

Museums, libraries, even cafés used to be silent spaces. They still are to some degree, but our multi-dimensional technology increasingly means public buildings are now designed to be multi-functional. Modern libraries do still have books, but serve more as a hub of different activities. Museums increasingly use moving images and sound. Sanctuaries such as churches are still an exception to the rule, but they are not always accessible, and in our secularized times we may hesitate to actually enter one. On the whole, I think we do ourselves a disservice by removing these islands of silence in the urban environment.

In really large cities silence is, of course, hard to come by, but with clever planning it's always possible to utilize even those small spaces that are left over after construction. New York's pocket parks are a good example of this. A small park in the middle of a city block is not silent in the auditory sense, but can still serve as a haven of sorts.

THE CHAPEL OF SILENCE
KAMPPI CHAPEL

Bearing in mind how silent sanctuaries are disappearing from our cities, where better to go next than to a place built solely to cater to this deeply felt need? In the heart of downtown Helsinki sits an unusual building, a small but towering chapel of wood that looks almost like a ship stranded in concrete. This is Kamppi Chapel (*shown opposite*), named for the part of town where it is located. Its unofficial name, however, is the "Chapel of Silence".

Although formally run by the Evangelical-Lutheran Church, the chapel – opened in 2012 – is open to all faiths. The direction of Mecca is marked on the floor, and there is also a section with cushions and stones representing Asian religions. Those wishing to meditate here are welcome.

The virtually soundproof chapel receives a constant stream of visitors, tourists and locals alike, presumably drawn here out of curiosity about this unusual place. With only one weekly scheduled devotion, this chapel is in a sense one of the most "inactive" in town.

Which, of course, is the whole point.

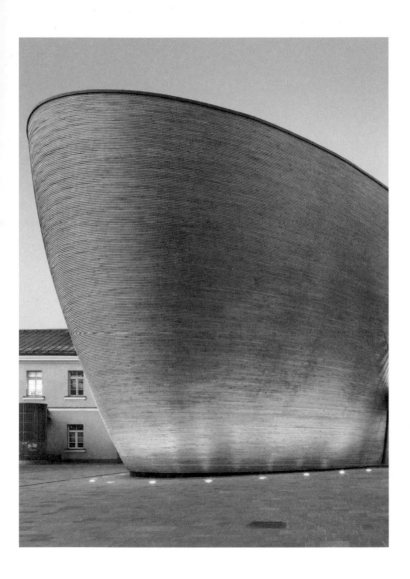

—

My Visit to the Chapel of Silence

A Test of Tolerance

—

The chapel, oblong and made entirely of wood, is smaller than it looks in photographs. A sign shows the rules: no speaking, no phones and no photography. The room is furnished with simple wooden benches. At the front is a small pulpit adorned with a tiny wooden cross. On the left side of it is a candle that never appears to flicker, on the right a minimalistic flower arrangement in a transparent vase, making it look from a distance as though the flowers are hovering in the air. The entire space is windowless save for the thinnest strip of glass, where the walls meet the ceiling. The day is overcast, but as I enter, a warm ray of sunshine emanates through the glass strip, illuminating the chapel with its vibrant light.

When I come in, there are about ten people seated here and there. Visitors are coming and going in a steady flow. The first impression that hits me is an odd sense of togetherness. What are we doing here, really? The chapel is so small and sparsely adorned that no one can pretend to stare at the architecture for very long – this is so obviously a place with a purpose. There is nowhere to hide: if you come here, ostensibly to see an example of lovely Finnish architecture, what you will encounter is an ode to silence.

I stay for 20 minutes, roughly estimating that the average time people spend here is 3 minutes. Everyone falls silent upon entering, and I'm positively surprised at how quickly people sit down and settle. (Not all, though. A group of adults sits down in front of me and one of them immediately picks up his phone and stays on it until his friends want to leave.)

During my visit, I experience three fleeting moments of

complete silence. They only last about ten seconds, but when they occur it feels as though everyone in the room is aware of it. The first time it happens I feel gratitude – I wasn't sure this place could actually deliver on its promise, and the silence feels like a gift. The second time I hold my breath without realizing it. The third time I get a sense (maybe just imagined) that we are all listening intently together. Time is suspended and hangs in the air like a drop of water. It will fall, of course, but those seconds before it does seem to matter more, and last longer, than seconds generally do.

Not for the Faint of Heart

Another interesting thing happens in those moments. It would appear that ten seconds is some kind of critical limit, because every time this deep silence occurs I can hear someone fidgeting a little, moving unnecessarily just to break it. A slight shifting in the seat, the faint rustling of a coat or a bag – when it happens the third time I'm positive that it's intentional. Nervous. Tense.

I would love to know what was going on in those people's minds just then. Did they break the silence involuntarily? Were they aware of breaking it or was it a gut reaction? Perhaps it was just a vague, unnamed sense of discomfort at a strange phenomenon?

The experience seems to take on more layers as I process it afterward. The contrast between the chapel and its very busy surroundings means that coming here is like being immediately whisked away to another place. As an experience it stands out in its oddness and beauty. It feels strange and – to use a word suitably removed from everyday language – hallowed.

I enjoyed it for my own sake,
but also realize that the most
thrilling aspect of this silence
for me is that it was experienced
together. The modern world
doesn't offer many opportunities
for a group of people to share
a time of unproductive silence.
A silence that may turn out to
be more revealing than any
number of words.

All profound things and emotions of things
are preceded and attended by silence

Herman Melville

Drop-in Silence – Same Space, Different Experiences

Intrigued by my experience at Kamppi Chapel, I talk to Nanna Helaakoski, the pastor and operative manager there, to find out more about why the chapel is so special.

What is the story behind the chapel?

The idea for this chapel originally came from Helsinki's Deputy Mayor at the time, Pekka Korpinen. He, in turn, was inspired by Rome, where every piazza has its own little church and locals are accustomed to popping in for just a few minutes with their bags of shopping in tow. The vision was to create something similar here, to offer people a respite from the loudness of daily life. As a concept the chapel is fairly unique and we've had some international interest.

Do people usually tell you what their experience was like?

Yes, frequently. It's clear from the feedback we get that different people perceive silence very differently. Sometimes two visitors will leave the chapel at the same time; one will say, "It was wonderfully quiet" and the other, "It wasn't quiet at all – and it was so annoying that someone took a photo!" The Finnish capacity for silence is comparatively high and our tolerance of noise in what is supposed to be a "quiet" place is consequently low. We get people from other parts of the country saying, "Oh, you need this here in the city, but we seek our silence in the forest." That's the traditional Finnish way. But we have lots of tourists here who may not come across silent spaces as readily, for whom a visit to the Kamppi chapel is a unique experience.

Some visitors tell us that the silence of the chapel made them cry, and although the reason may not be immediately obvious they feel it is a sign to dig deeper. Some people loved their visit, whereas others tell us it made them uncomfortable. They thought and felt things they didn't want to think and feel.

It's a silent space, but also very busy. How do you reconcile these opposites?

It's not always easy. There are lots of tourists visiting the chapel, especially around midday, and the door opening and closing all the time obviously makes it not all that silent. The regulars who use this chapel as a quiet place know this and tend to visit in the mornings or evenings.

People also have very different tolerance levels when it comes to silence. In my job as pastor, I encounter young people who really struggle with it. They often use music to wind down before bed – not classical, as you might expect, but up-tempo stuff. There is an aversion to silence that is bordering on the extreme. The chapel is not really a place that youngsters take to easily, especially when they arrive in groups. Being completely silent is for many so novel that even a few minutes are hard to manage. But I believe the experience can still be positive, as it is so different from everything else in their lives.

6

CREATING SILENCE

Saying nothing sometimes says the most

Emily Dickinson

NURTURING SILENCE
IDEAS AND INSPIRATION

In addition to seeking out nature and quiet city spaces, the notion is frequently put forward that silence is something we can create within us. That is all very well, but how exactly do we go about it? In this chapter, we take a look at some tangible, practical and potentially fun ways of cultivating inner silence, and we draw inspiration from two countries that have placed silence at the core of their way of life: Japan and Finland.

Any length of time spent walking the streets of a city, or visiting its shops and restaurants, is enough to convince me that the opportunities for silence are there. Perhaps not in the strictest sense, but sufficient for us to reap the refreshing effect that we long for. And yet after just a few hours of spontaneous field studies I can conclude that, on the whole, when a space opens up, we tend immediately to fill it with something.

I'm struck by how many people make or take calls over their solo lunch. I watch countless people – a majority – out running or walking amid sea breeze and birdsong, but they don't hear any of it through their headphones. Out on a stroll in nature with her baby in the pram, a mother is talking incessantly on the phone.

Sure, there is always the argument that there isn't enough time otherwise, that our lives are busy and packed with activity from dawn to dusk. And they are. But even so, why fill every occasion when we are alone with noise? Is it simply out of habit?

Going with the flow is always the easiest thing to do. There are any number of reasons why we may want to take the path of least resistance and, on the face of it, silence can seem like hard work – especially compared with chatting to someone or spending ten minutes scrolling social media. But once we get past that initial threshold, it is my belief that we will soon discover the healing, restorative properties of even just a little bit of silence.

But as we've already concluded, for those of us who are new to silence, there need to be paths we can take. What follows are some thoughts on creative ways of incorporating silence into our lives – ways that don't involve sitting still and just staring at a wall.

Silent Words – Books to the Rescue

This is a no-brainer. Disappearing between the covers of a book is one of the most satisfying silences there is. If it's a good one, our mind gets to rest from everyday worries and concerns and put all its focus elsewhere.

But uninterrupted reading is becoming rare. We have all heard the reports on decreasing attention spans that make reading and understanding longer texts more and more difficult. But what has been unlearned can be relearned – just leave the gadgets in another room and give the book your undivided attention. Your brain will thank you.

Framing Silence – Using Art to Create Inner Calm

Galleries are relatively silent places. There is usually no music playing, and visiting on a quiet day can feel a bit like entering a sanctuary. Most of the time there is an unspoken agreement to allow other people peace and quiet to enjoy the art. There is also something about the hushed, respectful way we tend to behave in the presence of art. Art appreciation is a private experience, and perhaps the reason many of us find it so cathartic is that it can act as a silent language for our own emotions.

Researcher Olga Lehmann (whom we first met on page 68) has not only worked on constructing a theory of silence, but

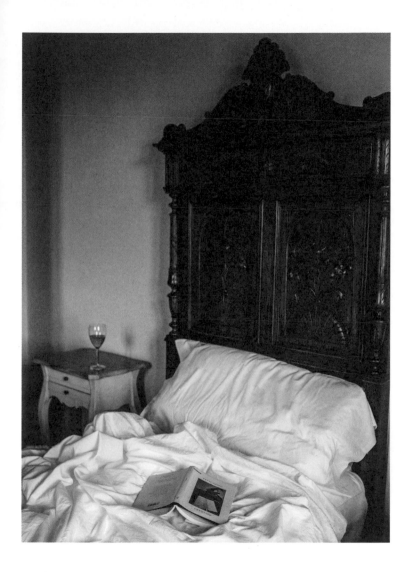

also investigates how art uses and relates to silence. "Art helps us express things we can't necessarily find words for," she says. "Putting words to feelings can be very difficult. We would often rather use music, art or poetry to help us get in touch with those feelings. If you do that – and combine art with silence – your art experience will be even stronger."

Art speaks to us, this much is true. But does the genre matter? Is there quiet versus loud art?

Considering that noise can be visual, art can indeed be loud. Many artists strive to awaken and perhaps shock us with their work and, when art communicates anguish, depression or dystopian visions, it may not exactly calm us down. But what is silent and what is loud depends on whom you ask – and regardless, art can, as Olga Lehmann says, serve as the silent catalyst we need to process our own emotions.

Quiet Views – How Colour and Design Affect Our Experience
When it comes to painters who can be said to have attempted to paint silence, my personal favourite is Vilhelm Hammershøi (1864–1916), a Danish artist who is still popular for his pared-down Nordic aesthetic and muted colour scheme. Hammershøi mostly painted interiors, and there is a quality to his style that seems to transport me into the very picture itself. If peopled at all, his domestic scenes usually

have just one person in them: often a woman, pictured with her back to the viewer. It is as if I can hear the backdrop of silence against which the everyday activities he depicts – sewing, reading – take place. The effect is one of stillness, growing on me gradually the longer I look.

This example also makes me wonder if current trends of minimalism and muted colours in interior design are another sign of our longing for silence. Life outside the home is busy, multi-coloured and often confusing, and we increasingly use our home as a shelter from the world. As the ultimate place of relaxation, it matters what the home looks like – perhaps more than ever.

I do think there are individual differences here. Some people don't seem very affected by living with piles of surplus stuff or bright colours, whereas others quickly find that it affects their wellbeing and concentration. What is certain is that many people have found that a visually uncluttered space can make an enormous difference to their peace of mind.

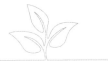

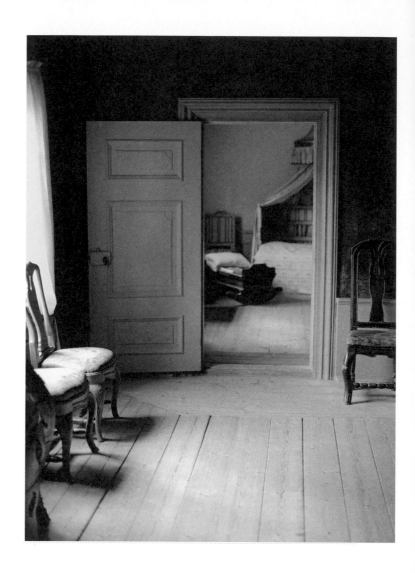

Mind Palace – The Calming Influence of Historic Places

Visiting sites where time seems to stand still, or has stopped altogether, and whose rooms carry a nice musty smell of years past and dust gathered, also creates a silence within me. It is a rich silence, heavy with memories and reminders of the lives that were once lived here. Such melancholy silences stay with me for a long time. When I need to relax, I let my mind go back to that room with the dusty books and ancient clock ticking away the hours, and it seems to lend me something of its deep stillness.

I've never heard anyone else suggesting that old places can be an excellent focal point of meditation, but for me that has certainly proved to be the case.

Time flies over us, but leaves
its shadow behind

Nathaniel Hawthorne

MINDFULLY MELLOW
MINDFULNESS WITH A TWIST

Most people nowadays are familiar with the concept of mindfulness. In its purest form, it centres on our breathing as a means of focusing and anchoring ourselves to the moment we are in. Those interested in developing their technique further have a plethora of books and techniques to choose from. But even as the practice becomes more commonplace, mindfulness still may not be everyone's cup of tea. If you find the idea of "practising" something just to keep you in the present a bit much, here are four alternative ideas on how to approach it.

1. Watch
If you suddenly became a witness to a crime and the police approached you to ask what you had seen and remembered, how helpful do you think you could be? That happened to me once, and much as I would have liked to impress the police officer with my razor-sharp powers of observation and photographic memory, my actual contribution was very modest. In my defence, this is how our brain works – constantly sorting and discarding impressions based on what we are likely to need. But the next time you are sitting idly on a train or bus, leave the phone aside and imagine yourself in spy school. What do you observe about the people you see? What general and specific conclusions can you draw about them?

If you are afraid to get caught staring, do the same with the landscape passing by. What do you notice? What catches your attention? Pretend you will be asked to describe it afterward. What would you say?

2. Slow down

Our thoughts strongly affect our bodies. Stressful thoughts tend to create hurried, rushed movements. When my stress levels soar, I employ a very simple technique that achieves the opposite: I force myself to do everything really slowly. Whether it's eating, writing, walking, doing the dishes or any other mundane task doesn't matter. It's not the action itself, but the slowness of it that sends the countersignals of calm that my brain so desperately needs. Before long, the action has begun working on my mind to help calm me down.

3. Speed up

There are few things I like so well as coming home from a run and just sitting still and staring into space for a while. Exercising or doing some kind of sport has a twofold effect on the mind: it helps us stay intently in the present, and it wearies the body to the point where an especially wonderful kind of silence emerges.

There is definitely less noise in my head afterward. It goes without saying that this effect can only be reached by making your time of training silent – no music or podcasts. You've been slightly hypnotized by the rhythm of your own breathing; now reap the benefits of the silent headspace that your effort has cleared for you.

4. Do stuff

In the words of Norwegian explorer and writer Erling Kagge:

Silence is about getting inside what you are doing. Experiencing rather than over-thinking. Allowing each moment to be big enough. Not living through other people and other things. Shutting out the world and fashioning your own silence whenever you run, cook food, have sex, study, chat, work, think of a new idea, read or dance.

How present are we really in this life of ours? I am endlessly fascinated by the idea that our everyday actions can become vehicles for inner silence. If silence forces us to be present in real and tangible ways, perhaps it can help us own the life we are actually living rather than waste time wishing for another.

Silence as a path to a truly independent and meaningful life – what's not to love?

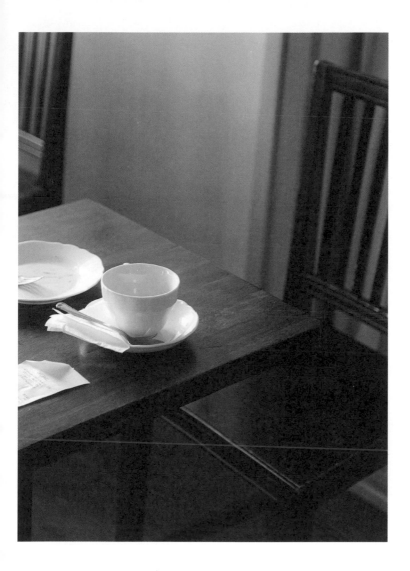

24 HOURS OF REST
DIGITAL SABBATH

The Sabbath – a full 24 hours of rest – is central to the Jewish faith. It used to be held in high regard in the Christian world as well, but commercial interests have eroded its importance in society. Nowadays we are used to everything being open "24/7" rather than "24/6". In a world driven by market interests and constant availability, there doesn't seem to be any reason that sounds even halfway valid for observing a day of rest.

Unfortunately. Because what if the religious command to observe a day of rest was always for our edification? In a world beset by FOMO (fear of missing out), those who keep the Sabbath increasingly feel it as a relief. For one day a week a fence is erected around daily life and, rather than limit space, it actually creates it.

What really happens if we turn our phones off for a day?

After I began to practise my own version of the Sabbath by staying away from social media for 24 hours, interesting things started to happen. The first few times, I was painfully aware of just how often my thoughts went to my phone; my hand would nervously hover over it before I remembered, at the last second, not to pick it up. I experienced recurring FOMO, which felt ridiculous, since I would be logging on again in a matter of hours.

And what did I discover when I did pick up the phone again? You guessed it: nothing much had happened. For certain, nobody had even noticed I was gone.

After a while I began looking forward to this one day of the week when some things would be off limits, instead giving space to others. On my self-imposed Sabbath I spend uninterrupted time being creative. I spend more time outside, and with family.

And I've begun to see this day as essential to my life. It acts as the hinge on which my week turns, contributing a rhythm that was missing from the "anytime, anywhere" mindset I used to have. Of course I don't need a command or permission slip to turn off my phone, but strangely enough it does make it easier. We are too afraid of rules – they do not always constrict.

Take a rest: a field that has rested
gives a beautiful crop

Ovid

SILENCE, PLEASE
FINLAND, WHERE SILENCE IS A VIRTUE
AS WELL AS A SELLING POINT

Most cultures perceive silence between people as awkward and something to be avoided at all costs. I live in Finland, which is a marked exception to the rule. Social silences here are so common and so accepted that foreigners sometimes get very unnerved. The underlying ethos is economy of language – if you haven't got anything worthwhile to say, then don't speak; don't throw out empty phrases just to keep the silence at bay. Silence acts as an invitation to sit down and just relax. Seen in its most positive light, this cultural oddity translates as social generosity extended from one person to another.

It is true that silence in a group can also feel morose and at times depressive – and sometimes it is. Not all silences are healthy, even in Finland. But broadly speaking, once you start to relax into this communal silence it dawns on you what it really is, namely a lack of pressure. This sense of being welcome as you are, whether or not you have anything valuable to contribute, is something I have not felt to the same extent anywhere else.

But where does this love of silence come from? Finns like to think it is something of a by-product of centuries of life spent in a largely empty country, with great swaths of genuine wilderness still available today – not to mention a

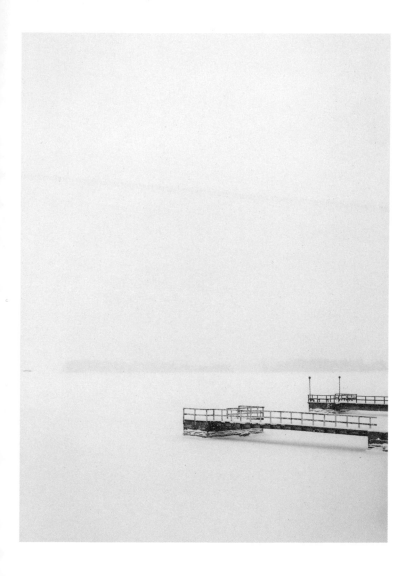

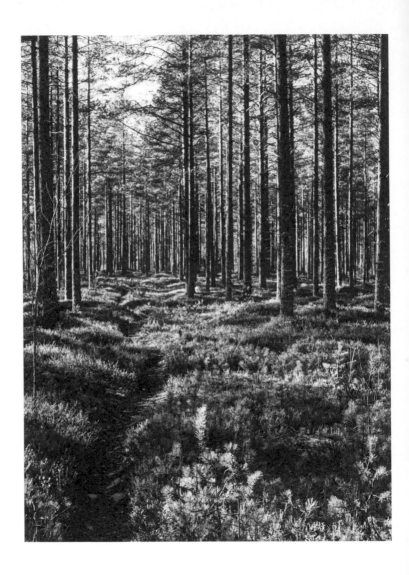

lot of personal space. Finns still nurture a close and loving relationship with nature and love to spend long stretches of time in little cabin hideaways. Hiking in the northern wilderness is an annual tradition for many, and most Finns regularly spend time in the forest, foraging for berries or just enjoying its peace and quiet.

Aside from informing its culture, silence in all its forms is widely appreciated in Finland. In 2011, the Finnish Tourist Board latched on to this and launched a marketing campaign that had the slogan "Silence, Please". In using silence as a marketing tool, they sought to entice people to visit the country and experience for themselves the beauty of silence.

In the years since, "silence tourism" has become a global niche where Finland fits very nicely. Making use of an increasingly rare natural resource that happens to be bountiful here has proved a success. Weary urbanites often have silence at the top of their holiday wish list and – what's more – are willing to pay for it. Being sparsely populated with quiet people, Finland is ready to deliver.

HOT IN HERE
SILENCE AND THE SAUNA

Another place where social silence is cultivated is in that quintessential Finnish sanctuary, the sauna.

Finns generally like their saunas hot, between 80° and 120°C (175° and 250°F), and the heat is very conducive to silence. Breathing becomes slower and more deliberate, and there is also the aspect of feeling muscles and joints relaxing – much like in a hot bath – to the point of peaceful bliss bordering on sleepiness.

My thoughts run slowly in the sauna. It is actually a very meditative place, and even when you are enjoying it with friends, not much is said.

The intimacy of the sauna means it also has a reputation for being exclusive. In the corporate world it used to be said it was in the all-male sauna sessions, not the boardroom, that business deals were *really* made, obviously excluding any women who had vested interests to defend. This kind of "sauna culture" is increasingly a thing of the past, however – not least because these days businesswomen are more likely to don a towel and join in.

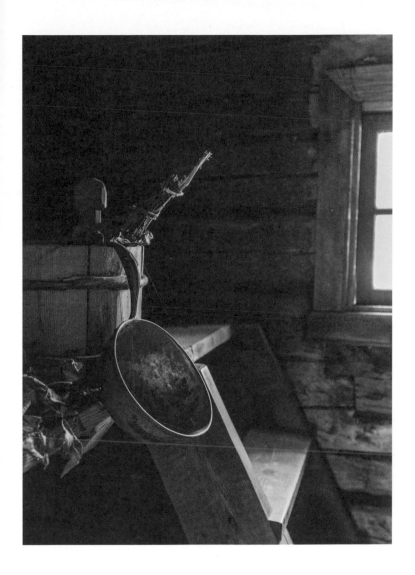

Honouring the Silence – How Japanese Culture Thrives on Quiet

There is one culture where silence is a key component of all aspects of life from personal refreshment to traditional rituals: Japan. Whether it's relaxing in a traditional bath, savouring tea in silence with strangers or just taking a balanced approach to life, Japanese culture has stillness at its core. To understand more about the role silence plays in life in Japan I speak to Hiroko Matsuyama, a Tokyo-based writer who specializes in writing about Japanese culture for the English-speaking world. Together with her photographer partner she also runs a Japanese culture website called PATTERNZ.

The Japanese tea ceremony is characterized by silence, slow, deliberate movements, the equality of everyone present and an intense focus on the moment. Where does it originate, and is it something that Japanese people regularly take part in?

The habit of drinking tea is deeply connected to Zen Buddhism, as Buddhist priests first introduced tea for medicinal use. Wealthy merchants embraced it, followed by the Samurai class, and in the end regular people also started drinking it for sheer enjoyment. Since the goal of practising Zen is to be aware of one's Buddha nature by reaching a state of enlightenment, the tea ceremony is a vehicle for achieving that stillness. In Zen, the saying is that you can clear the clutter in your mind and achieve stillness by sitting up straight. We see this in the Zen posture of seated meditation called *zazen*.

Not every Japanese person regularly takes part in a tea ceremony. However, a certain number practise it regularly and enjoy the benefits. It is very common for young people to get a chance to engage with it, as most schools have a tea ceremony club.

Each tea ceremony is unique: people are able to appreciate and enjoy the moment for its uniqueness. It can't happen the same way again, or anywhere else.

A hanging scroll in the tea ceremony room indicates a subject of the day. Signifying something through abstract and indirect expression is characteristic of Japanese culture, and the tea ceremony is no exception.

One can say that performing and participating in a tea ceremony can cultivate your sense of focus, stillness and unity.

Traditional Japanese gardens are built around silent appreciation of nature, especially perhaps the Zen garden with its carefully planned structure. When you visit a Japanese garden, what is your expectation? Do you come just to relax or is there a deeper purpose to it?

I'm very familiar with those gardens since my grandfather built one in front of his house. As a young child I didn't appreciate it so much, as I preferred more natural gardens with flowers. But once you understand the codes behind it, the meaning behind the placement of everything, you appreciate and enjoy the Japanese garden more. Everything has meaning, such as stones signifying the sacred mountain or specific animals. You can think over the meanings and what the creator wanted to express with his garden.

Whether you wish to relax or try to understand the significance of each object in a Japanese garden, you will notice how the garden helps to clear and calm your mind. It has a certain order and intention behind it.

It seems to me that many aspects of Japanese culture tend to cultivate a sense of quiet focus. Aside from the gardens and the tea ceremony, I'm thinking of the baths, but also of art forms such as calligraphy, origami and bonsai. What role would you say that silence plays in Japanese culture?

We have a saying: "Silence is golden". We esteem reserved people as highly as those who can express themselves eloquently. All of the practices you mention make you focus on what you are doing in the moment. They let you be aware of your senses instead of the ideas in your head, which helps you connect yourself to your core rather than to something you can capture with your mind.

Japan is a densely populated country with large, busy cities. What do ordinary Japanese people do to find peace of

*mind in the midst of bustling urban life? Do they experience
a clash between an older, calmer way of life and the fast
pace of today?*

Everyone has their own method of creating moments that
soothe the mind. It is true, though, that it's getting harder
to experience a quiet focus these days, as the mobile
phone has become our second skin and our brains tend
to overflow with information from outside.

Quite a few people seek out meditation, any sort of
meditation that suits them. Yoga is also always popular
here, especially among women.

Even if you don't practise meditation or yoga, people
who have access to nature or have a pet are fortunate
in that they can more easily remind themselves to feel
rather than think and constantly try to make a meaning
out of everything.

7

...AND THE REST IS SILENCE – A THOUGHTFUL SUMMARY

Let silence be the art you practise

Rumi

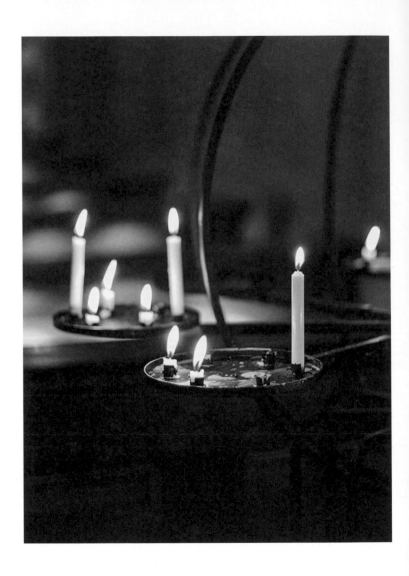

INTO SILENCE
NOTES FROM THE PATH

Silence – enigmatic, scary, rich, full of risk and possibility – is a fascinating force. There is so much more to say about it than I could have imagined. In this final chapter, I try to summarize what writing this book has meant to me and what surprising discoveries I've made in the process. These parting words also contain something of a nudge and a plea.

Reading about silence, spending time in silence, pondering the different qualities of silence...over the time it has taken for this book to emerge, I have been doing a lot of these things. Given the nature of the topic, I felt from the start that I also wanted to try living differently for a season. Cut down on the amount of sounds and social media, as well as time spent online or watching television or films. I've not gone completely without any of these, but I have lived differently. And it's been good.

So what do I take away from all this? Has it changed me, and if so, how?

It has. For instance, I increasingly think of silence as being quantifiable. Silence has gone from being a vague concept, about as easy to pin down as fog, to something more solid and tangible. I can go in search of it. I can create it myself. But this solidification of silence comes, I think, from being able to tell how increasing amounts of it affect me. It is as if I myself am being solidified.

So much of what is necessary in life requires us to clear a certain amount of space. In order for me to be fully present in my relationships with people, the core of my being needs silence. If chaos and noise prevail, I lack the necessary focus to come out of myself and meet others. However, this requires meeting myself first, without distractions, noise, other voices and impulses. I do believe that one of the main reasons for the anguish that so many people experience now is our inability to do just that. We aren't used to it, and we aren't taught how.

In a world where it is possible to distract ourselves quite literally from the cradle to the grave, is it any wonder that we are anxious?

Speech is silver, silence is gold

Swedish proverb

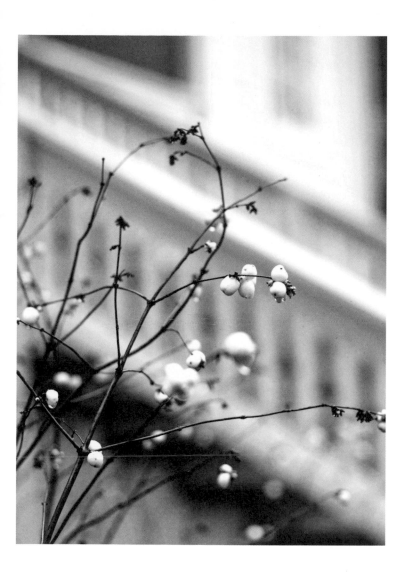

LESSONS IN SILENCE
WHAT I'VE LEARNED THAT STANDS OUT

What follows are my most important insights, crystallized into four calls to action.

1. Understand that constant distraction has consequences

A lack of silence hinders our thinking, most importantly our capacity for long-term planning and for *predicting the consequences of our actions*. This is a really important insight. A constantly interrupted train of thought is, after a while, no longer a train but a series of separate carriages going nowhere. It doesn't take much to understand the dire consequences of an entire world of constantly distracted individuals making decisions for the future. (I fear we may be seeing some fallout already.) But with a concentrated effort to get our superb thinking machines back on track, we would doubtless also see a positive ripple effect.

2. Embrace the difficulty of silence

There is no getting away from the fact that silence is a shape-shifter that can feel restful one day and alarming the next. Spending more time making friends with silence will obviously help a lot. But even so I strongly believe that we need to embrace the duality inherent in silence, that it can be *both awkward and good for us at the same time*.

Taking on board the notion that silence needs practice can be helpful here. When we train for an athletic goal, it's not the individual training sessions that matter, but quantity and repetition. Little by little, we can become skilled at embracing silence, hopefully to the point where it becomes second nature and something we wouldn't want to live without.

3. Explore the power of shared silence

I'd never before considered that silence could have a communal aspect, probably since the very idea of organized, shared silence lasting longer than a minute is so extremely rare. It flies in the face of most of our ideals of efficiency, action and momentum. It seems, on the face of it, extremely unproductive. But silence does appear to promote peace. And with silence as the baseline, our brains receive a much-needed boost to both focus and efficiency.

Perhaps precisely because silent moments are so rare and so hard to come by - and with so very few role models to lead the way - schools and other institutions of education could play a really important role by implementing a time of silence at the start of each day. Even just a few minutes could be enough to decrease tensions and disruptions and create an increase in efficiency over the course of the day. Thinking of it this way, it seems hard to believe it isn't already a fixture in our society. However, there is nothing stopping you and me from implementing it in our lives, starting tomorrow.

4. Allow your mind the space it needs to work

When it comes to distractions, I am my own worst enemy (as I believe you may be yours). Learning about the default mode network has attuned me to a particular feeling of calm thoughtfulness that, for me at least, signals its presence.

Writing a book has proved an excellent lab for testing this hypothesis. All creative work, after all, requires a certain faith in growth – things don't come out fully formed but need space and peace to develop. The more time the brain is allowed to spend in the default mode, the more creative it becomes.

I think part of the reason why we distract ourselves is that our brains are capable of such a lot. Forcing them to focus on just one thing at a time – no scrolling the phone while watching a film, for instance – can, at least on days when we feel well rested and energetic, actually feel like underusing our mental capacity. But the restlessness that comes from technological multi-tasking is an insidious, stealthily growing thing. We may not even notice it before insomnia has hit.

So here's my new truth: multi-tasking is not our friend, it only poses as one.

I'm now trying to relearn how to single-task. I won't deny it is difficult at times, but what keeps me going is the belief that I'm doing myself a huge favour in the long run. Better cognition, attention span, memory, creativity, efficiency and peace of mind really *do* attract me more than another hour spent distracting myself.

Silence is the element in which great things fashion themselves together

Thomas Carlyle

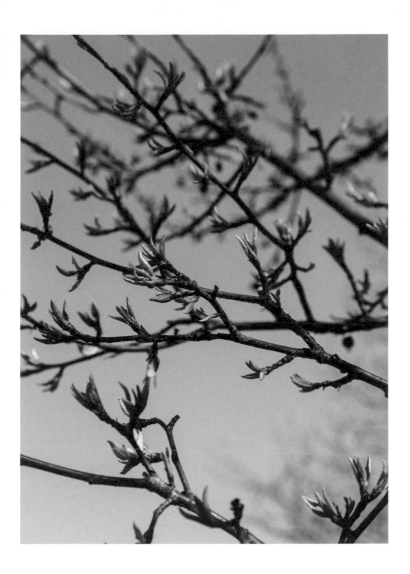

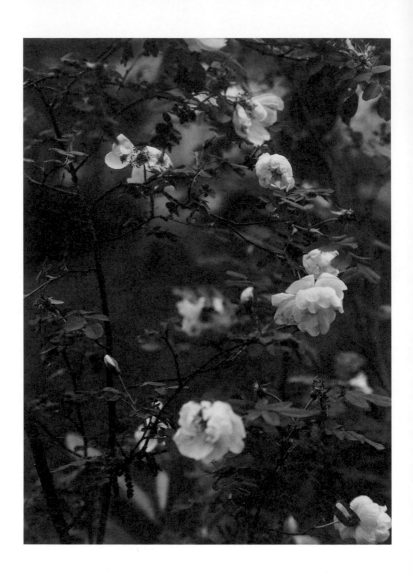

THE FUTURE IS SILENT
TAKING THE FIRST STEPS

If I've learned anything at all about the challenges of this technologically driven world, it is this: we need to take charge of our lives. If we don't, *something else will.*

Going with the flow has never been so easy. Yes, technology has brought us wonderful inventions and gloriously easy access to knowledge, enjoyment and even other people. But (and you knew there was a but) – it's threatening to take over our lives to the point of ruining our health, our relationships and even the cognitive functions of our brains. The problem of always living within a virtual bubble of image and sound is that the world outside starts to feel increasingly foreign.

We can't always affect the noise around us, but we can often do a lot more about the kind of noise we ourselves choose to generate. I believe we would do well to clear some space. To think, feel, be, communicate and engage with others, make better decisions, live from a place of calm – for the improvement of just about every aspect of life.

If you agree with me, why not try some of the ideas in this book for yourself? Start your day with a couple of quiet minutes. Go for a silent walk. Gaze at a favourite painting. Perhaps you will find one or two things that stick. Chances are, you won't regret it.

REFERENCES

Chapter 1: The Sound of Silence
Page 16: https://en.m.wikipedia.org/
wiki/4'33

Chapter 3: Numbing Noise, Soothing Silence
Page 54: http://www.euro.who.int/__data/
assets/pdf_file/0008/136466/e94888.pdf
Page 56: *Psychological Science* (Sept
2002, Vol. 13, No. 5, pp 469-74)
Page 56: https://www.apa.org/
monitor/2011/07-08/silence
Page 58: https://jamanetwork.com/
journals/jama/fullarticle/186427
Page 61: https://www.ncbi.nlm.nih.gov/
pmc/articles/PMC1860853/
Page 61: https://www.researchgate.net/
publication/259110014_Is_silence_golden_
Effects_of_auditory_stimuli_and_their_
absence_on_adult_hippocampal_
neurogenesis

Chapter 4: A Silent Mind
Page 66: https://science.sciencemag.org/
content/345/6192/75 Science 04 Jul 2014:
Vol. 345, Issue 6192, pp. 75-77
Page 74: https://psycnet.apa.org/
record/2014-52280-001
Page 74: https://www.psychologytoday.
com/intl/blog/the-squeaky-wheel/201501/
how-cellphone-use-can-disconnect-
your-relationship

Page 74: *Helsingin Sanomat* (Antti Tiainen)
21 May 2019: https://www.hs.fi/teknologia/
art-2000006112510.html
Page 80: https://www.kyrkpressen.fi/
aktuellt/57499-pa-retreat-ar-tystnaden-
beloningen-och-utmaningen.html

Chapter 5: Finding Silence
Page 91: https://journals.sagepub.com/doi/
abs/10.1111/j.1467-9280.2008.02225.x
Page 91: https://journals.sagepub.com/doi/
abs/10.1177/1087054708323000
Page 91: https://www.ncbi.nlm.nih.gov/
pubmed/22840583
Page 91: https://www.ncbi.nlm.nih.gov/
pubmed/21996763
Page 91: https://www.tandfonline.com/doi/
abs/10.1080/02827580701262733#.
U0VZHOZdXz0
Page 93: https://www.ncbi.nlm.nih.gov/
pmc/articles/PMC3393816/
Page 93: https://www.ncbi.nlm.nih.gov/
pmc/articles/PMC2793341/

Chapter 6: Creating Silence
Page 128: Kagge, Erling, *Silence in the Age
of Noise*, (London: Penguin, 2018,
translated from the Norwegian). Quoted by
permission of the author.

All websites accessed June 2019

PICTURE CREDITS

Geordie Stewart 25.

iStock Andrey Danilovich 32; bruev 95; Marc Lechanteur 101; Matti Salminen 137; Pieter-Pieter 31; ReaTiina 134; Sebastien Lemyre 50.

Joanna Nylund 4-5, 6, 12, 17, 20, 23, 28-29, 36, 49, 59, 60, 63, 69, 72, 81, 85, 92, 97, 102, 105, 124, 129, 144, 147, 150, 153, 154.

Marko Huttunen 109.

Pexels Aleksandr Slobodianyk 110-113; Evie Shaffer 10-11; Johannes Plenio 76-79; Magda Ehlers 40-45; Pixabay 52-53, 86-87, 116-117; Snapwire 64-65.

Pixabay Kanenori 142-143.

Rebecca Skye Watson 9, 35, 89, 121, 133.

Shutterstock LuckyStep 39.

INDEX

ACKNOWLEDGEMENTS

My heartfelt thanks to everyone I interviewed or consulted during the writing of this book, for your generosity and wonderful insights: Dr Olga Lehmann, Geordie Stewart, Milo Dahlmann, Hiroko Matsuyama, Pirkko-Liisa Schulman, Emelie Wikblad, Nanna Helaakoski, Helsinki's Quaker Community, Michael Freund, Elsa Kaijala.

Thank you my dear friend Rebecca Skye Watson for letting me include some of your beautiful photographs!

I'd also like to thank Jussi Kiilamo for the inspiration, and the whole team at Octopus Books for believing in the book and being such a joy to work with.

The greatest of love and thanks to Johnny; you are truly the wind beneath my wings.

The Eternal One, whose first language is silence: you have my words and my silences.